PAIN:
Why It Hurts
Where It Hurts
When It Hurts

Other Books by Richard Stiller

The Best Policy
Broken Promises
Commune on the Frontier
The Felix Factor
The Love Bugs
Queen of Populists
The Spy, the Lady, the Captain and the Colonel

PAIN:
Why It Hurts
Where It Hurts
When It Hurts

BY RICHARD STILLER

THOMAS NELSON INC., PUBLISHERS

NASHVILLE • NEW YORK

First Edition

Library of Congress Cataloging in Publication Data

Stiller, Richard.
   Pain: why it hurts, where it hurts, when it hurts.

   Summary: Includes chapters on headaches, backaches, women and pain,
drugs as pain control, acupuncture analgesia, and hypnosis and biofeedback.
   1. Pain.   [1. Pain]   I. Title. [DNLM: 1. Pain—Popular works. WL700
S857p]
RB127.S75   616'.047   75–6522
ISBN 0–8407–6430–8

Acknowledgments

I am indebted to Dr. Ronald Melzack, Department of Psychology, McGill University, Dr. Peter Sterling, Department of Anatomy, University of Pennsylvania School of Medicine, and Dr. B. Berthold Wolff, Department of Medicine, New York University School of Medicine, for reading the manuscript of this book prior to publication and for offering critical comments.

I wish also to thank Dr. Alan C. Hymes, Department of Surgery, University of Minnesota, Dr. Don M. Long, Department of Neurological Surgery, The Johns Hopkins Hospital, and Dr. Arthur Taub, Neurological Research Laboratory, Yale University School of Medicine, for reading and commenting on the chapter on electroanalgesia; and Dr. James Burke, Manchester, New Hampshire, and Dr. Leon Feinstein, Port Chester, New York, dental practitioners, for reading and commenting on the chapter on dental pain.

I am grateful to the following for their help in the preparation of this book: Prof. James Freeman, Department of Anthropology, San Jose State University, California; Dr. Jean E. Johnson, Center for Health Research, Wayne State University, Michigan; Dr. Herbert F. Spasser, Department of Endodontics, New York University College of Dentistry; and Dr. J.

Lawrence Pool, Professor Emeritus of Neurological Surgery, Columbia-Presbyterian Medical Center.

All of the above contributed to whatever merit this book possesses; responsibility for errors of interpretation or misstatements of fact is mine alone.

RICHARD STILLER

Contents

Chapter 1

A Part of Life

From its very beginning life is touched by pain: a mother's pain of stretched and tearing tissues as she labors to give birth, her baby's lusty cry of pain as it knocks on the door.

It is even possible that late in pregnancy the unborn baby feels pain while still in the womb. A fetus will pull its leg away from a pinprick. But the womb is a silent place, and fetuses have not yet made their complaints heard.

Although newborn babies cry, it was assumed for many years that they did not feel pain because they could not (or did not) complain of a specific hurt in a specific place. So anesthesia during surgery was considered unnecessary for infants.

But they do feel pain, although their reactions are hard to evaluate. On the first day of an infant's life, its physical reaction to a pinch or a pinprick is relatively slow. About half a second passes before the infant jerks or pulls away, another two to three seconds before it cries. As the days and months go by, that time lag shortens.

By the time a child is six, it responds almost instantaneously to an electric shock one eighth as powerful as the shock needed to cause a delayed reaction when the child was one day old. More significant—the child knows exactly where the hurt is. It has learned an important part of life—how to react to and deal with pain.

Dealing with pain is difficult because it is a complicated experience. Describing pain is as hard as putting the hurt into words. Pain is a sensation, but not *just* a sensation, not a sixth sense added on to the senses of sight, smell, sound, taste, and touch. These five primary sensations bring news of the outside world into the brain. They tell the individual what's happening, where it's at, how it smells, what it feels like.

The pain sensation not only brings the bad news of hurt. It also triggers defensive action. A baby blinks its eyes against a grain of sand, pulls away from a hot radiator. An animal flinches from a blow, turns its head toward the hurt. These automatic reactions are regulated by the brainstem, the lower part of the brain that controls involuntary actions (breathing, heartbeat), and by the spinal cord. These reactions—they used to be called instinctive—require no thought.

Such automatic reactions requiring no thought raise a question. Are they "pain"? If a frog is dissected in the laboratory so that its brain is removed, its leg will still twitch away from a needle jab. Does the frog "feel" anything?

Probably not. A sensation must be *perceived*, in order to be felt as pain, and the only organ capable of perception is the brain. Without a brain—or with a brain that is not functioning—nothing is "felt." When a stroke destroys one side of the brain, no sensation can be felt on the opposite side of the body.

Another special quality of pain is that it forces an expression through noise, or vocalization: a baby cries; an animal whimpers or howls; an adult groans.

Human pain is different from animal pain in that the thoughtful, conscious reaction of being hurt is triggered in the cerebrum, the topmost part of the brain. This aspect of pain, the conscious reaction to it, is the most difficult to understand, and in fact we do not yet understand it. It is in the covering layer of the cerebrum, its cortex, that we react consciously to pain—*really* feel it. Here, where the power to think exerts its decisive influence and makes us human, we deal with pain in accordance with our memory, knowledge, and personality.

A man feels pain. He remembers that the last time he had such a pain it was caused by appendicitis. He also knows that it is not considered "manly" to pay too much attention to pain, and especially to make complaining noises. Does this new pain mean another attack of appendicitis? A simple case of gas? A heart attack? Cancer? Will he have to have an operation? Should he give in and seek help or bear his pain "manfully"? Will the doctor laugh at him? Will his wife be sympathetic or will she ridicule him? Should he worry? Will it go away?

The pain is in his abdomen, but all these pain processes take place in his brain, and mostly in the topmost part of his brain, the eighth-of-an-inch-thick cerebral cortex. Here, in fact, is where the pain message is received and pain will be perceived. The way one perceives pain has a great deal to do with the pain itself—how long it lasts, how bad it feels, how one deals with it.

Pain is a very special part of life, like no other part. It mixes unpleasant sensations, defensive reactions, noisy expressions, and intellectual and emotional circumstances. It is complicated, intricate, and mysterious.

And very personal.

Try telling someone about how it feels when you hurt. Can you communicate it accurately?

This is the problem a doctor faces when he tries to diagnose a patient's pain. The patient says, "It hurts around the chest. Especially when I lift my arm. Sometimes it's like a stabbing knife. Other times it feels dull and aching."

"What do these words mean?" the doctor thinks. "Do they mean the same thing to the patient they mean to me? Do they mean the same as the same words used by another patient?"

The vocabulary of pain is long and confusing, varies from person to person, and is unreliable. An imaginative, articulate patient may paint his pain in vivid detail. A less verbal person finds that the words come hard to his lips. Is his pain the less?

When one attempts to describe pain, one finds how inaccurate the description of it as a "sensation" is. It is, in fact, many *kinds* of sensations and may be described as beating, stabbing, crushing, nauseating, dragging, nagging, excruciating, annoying, rhythmic, radiating, pricking, itching, etc.

In an effort to understand and classify the terms people use to describe pain, two Canadian pain researchers asked two hundred individuals—men and women, doctors and patients, students and college graduates—to pick the words they thought described pain. The researchers discovered more than one hundred, ranging from "agonizing" to "violent," and divided them into fourteen different pain categories. Nine of these categories described different qualities of the sensation such as its location, relation to time, pressure, and stretching. Four described emotional reactions to pain. The last category sorted out and evaluated the degree of pain as ranging from bearable to unbearable.

Even pain researchers do not agree that the single word "pain" is a sufficiently precise label. The late Sir Thomas Lewis, a distinguished British physician, described two types of pain and thought that the differences between them were so great that the use of one word for both was "unsafe."

Sir Thomas distinguished between what he called skin pain and deep pain. The first, caused by injury to the surface of the body, was a kind of pricking sensation that did not last long, followed by a more lasting, burning feeling. The dull, deep pain felt in injured or diseased muscles, joints, bones, and inner tissues and organs was, he suggested, much more painful.

He also divided skin or surface pain into two stages: first a fast, flashing sensation, followed by a second slower, longer-lasting, more intense pain. Each stage, he said, may be carried by different pain nerves. And he added that some part of the body (head, shoulders, back) apparently felt only the first, fast pain, while other parts felt both stages.

Using our cerebral cortex, we evaluate and consider pain, make judgments about it, put labels on it, and decide where it comes from and what to do for it. This uniquely human organ of intelligence can be misled, however. The very word "pain" comes from the Latin word for punishment. Clearly, our ancestors' cerebrums "explained" pain as a penalty for wickedness, not as a complicated sensation with important defensive qualities.

Ironically, the very organ that perceives pain for the rest of the body cannot feel pain itself. A knife or a cancer in brain tissue does not hurt. But fortunately, the brain and spinal cord, which make up our central nervous system, and the nerve fibers that make up our other nervous systems, can and do sound the pain alarm when the body is threatened. Without this early warning alarm system, we would have no defense against attacks by heat, puncture, infection, blows, or other dangers.

Chapter 2

A World Without Pain

There are people for whom pain is *not* a part of life. They do not feel it, anywhere in their bodies, although they feel all other sensations. A person with this strange analgesia —absence of pain—can feel the touch of a feather, the kiss of a breeze, pressure, heat, and cold— but not cuts, burns, tears, or punctures of the skin or other tissues.

Less than one hundred such individuals have been reported in medical literature, but their puzzling condition is far more interesting and important to pain researchers than their numbers indicate. If their analgesia can ever be understood and explained, much that remains a mystery about pain and how to relieve it will also be revealed.

One eight-year-old English girl developed this condition after an inflammation of the lining of the brain caused by the viral disease encephalitis. She absentmindedly pulled out all but nine of her teeth without noticing it. A few years later, while in the hospital, she poked both her eyes out of their sockets. She was afraid she would be punished for this, and so she said they "fell out" while she was asleep. She scratched her cheek so hard she drew blood.

This girl could feel no pain, although she could feel the difference between the sharp and the blunt end of a pin. Doctors were unable, after careful examination, to find any physical abnormality to explain her indifference to pain.

Another girl, the daughter of a Canadian physician, felt no pain from birth—a condition known as congenital analgesia. Once, when she chewed her food, she bit off the tip of her tongue without being aware of it. To look out a high window, she knelt on a hot radiator, suffered severe burns—and did not know it. Electric shocks did not hurt her. In addition, she never sneezed, coughed, or gagged. Her eyelids did not blink at the approach of a foreign object. When she was very little, she poked a stick into her nose and pierced a nostril.

This girl, probably because her father was a doctor, was studied carefully all her life and is probably the most written-about case of congenital analgesia in medical history. She grew up to be entirely normal in all other respects, and went off to college. Since she never knew when she was putting undue pressure on her joints, she suffered from many bone fractures, and she had many serious infections, because she was never warned by pain or discomfort that she was sick. And so she did not live very long. She died in her twenties; only during the last month of her life did she feel any discomfort.

After her death her body was carefully autopsied. Nothing abnormal was discovered. To this day pain researchers, evaluating her strange and tragic life, suspect that she had some undetected brain or nerve defect, something too small to be seen at that time under the microscope.

For it is the nervous system—the brain, the spinal cord, and the peripheral nerves that branch out from the spinal cord to outlying parts of the body—that carries pain messages. In the following chapters, and especially in Chapter 6, we will see how this nervous system receives and reacts to pain signals or stimuli. But we can say something now about the three neurological processes that contribute to pain. (Neurological processes are processes of the nervous system.)

The *feeling* or *sensation* of pain is the result of the action of nerve fibers leading from the skin and organs of the body to the spinal cord, which is itself a thick collection of many nerve fibers running like a cable from the lower part of the body up into the brain.

Automatic reactions to pain, or reflexes—such as pulling away from a hot object or blinking an eye at a speck of dust near the eyeball—require no thought or will. These reactions are regulated by the spinal cord and do not necessarily (although they sometimes can) travel up to the brain. The brain can influence these reactions, however.

Conscious reactions to pain, or the *perception* of pain—Why does my eye burn? Does that chest pain mean I should see a doctor? That pain is coming from my big toe, right foot—take place in the brain. It is in and through various parts of the brain, a massive blob of nerve tissue, that everything that happens to the body—including pain—is regulated, evaluated, and reacted to.

Why do these otherwise normal individuals fail to feel pain signals warning of life-threatening dangers? Some researchers speculate that there may be invisible damage to the nerve fibers that carry pain signals. This damage may have been caused by one or another nerve disease.

A suspected cause of congenital analgesia is the hereditary disease called familial dysautonomia. Its victims are almost always children of Jewish descent. Usually, in this rare condition the child is insensitive to or feels no pain; yet sometimes, he or she may feel intense pain. Children with familial dysautonomia also lack common motor reflexes; they have difficulty, for example, shedding tears.

These strange cases provide evidence that pain serves a useful function. All these patients sicken and die because they are unprotected. Without pain, living organisms, from humans on down the scale to the most primitive forms of animal life, cannot survive because they do not avoid injury or react to its threats.

Pain is a protective sensation. Any organism with a nervous system can feel the unpleasant stimuli that we humans call pain. Plants have no nervous system, and cannot feel pain, although they do react to harmful stimuli in their own way. All forms of animal life have nervous systems, although these differ from one class, such as mammals, to another, such as insects.

The most protective reaction to pain sensation is the automatic reflex—the jerk of a cut finger, the retreat and flight of a hurt animal. This mechanism probably developed first as living creatures evolved. We humans carry this elementary reflex with us from our earliest prehistoric days.

But of all the animals only humans appear to react in a complicated, conscious way to pain—to think about it, to perceive it. Only humans have the large, highly developed cerebral cortex necessary for this reaction. Chimpanzees and other great apes have small cerebral cortices; lower animals have just the beginnings of a cortex; birds, fish, and insects have none at all. Our cerebral cortex enables us to think, speculate, remember, worry—about pain as well as about everything else. It even enables us to think about thinking.

Pain signals travel from the outer nerve fibers into the spinal cord and up the cord, ending in a part of the brain —deep in its center—called the thalamus. The thalamus is an extraordinarily complicated relay switching station which transmits nerve impulses to other parts of the brain, including the cerebrum, and also responds to impulses *from* the cerebrum.

The message passes in some as-yet-unknown way from the thalamus to the cerebral cortex for final disposition. The cortex reacts to pain in many ways. It makes decisions: sending us to the doctor, to the drugstore for a pain-killer, to a witch doctor for a magic charm, to prayer for relief. Or it causes us to worry.

When a person drinks too much liquor, he describes himself as "feeling no pain." True enough. The effect of liquor is to turn off the cerebral cortex. That is why it relaxes the drinker. When the cortex is not working as usual, we don't seem to notice—don't "feel" the pain.

The existence of the cerebral cortex in humans complicates pain and makes it much more than a "primitive protective mechanism." Pain can also be a curse.

Some years ago the French surgeon Rene Leriche suggested that pain in humans was at best an ineffective alarm signal, at worst a calamity. He said: "The majority of diseases, even the most serious, attack us without warning. When pain develops . . . it is too late."

Heart disease, one of our three major killers, often strikes without warning pain. Even when there is a pain warning, it often comes close to the actual heart attack, and death follows within minutes. When there is a good deal of time before death, it is not always easy for the victim (or for the doctor) to interpret chest or arm or shoulder pain correctly as heart disease pain.

High blood pressure is an important cause of heart disease and of stroke, a second major killer. There is no warning pain before a stroke. One of the problems in treating high blood pressure is that people don't know they have it unless a doctor measures it and tells them. Even then, they often resist taking necessary medication and other protective steps because they feel no discomfort.

People pay more attention to sunburn or athlete's foot, because these ailments hurt, than they do to high blood pressure, which doesn't.

A third major killer is cancer. Cancer of the brain produces no pain. Neither do *the early stages* of most other cancers. By the time cancer hurts, it is often too late. Then, long after the pain can serve as a useful warning, cancer produces the most excruciating of tortures.

There are other major diseases that contribute to early death or disability but do not send any early warning pain signals. Diabetes, glaucoma, and such degenerative diseases as multiple sclerosis, muscular dystrophy, and scleroderma are some of these.

Why is it that relatively simple, even minor, and rarely fatal injuries—cuts, bruises, blows, burns, fractures—send us quick and agonizing pain signals, while the mass murderers do not?

One hypothesis (the scientist's name for what is hoped will be an intelligent guess) is that it is because the "primitive" protective sensation of pain developed in our nervous system very early in the timetable of evolution, when our brain had a thalamus but little or no cerebral cortex. The cortex—that organ which makes us human by enabling us to think and to possess a conscience, a sense of what is right and wrong—was the last part of our body to evolve.

We humans have basically not changed physically since our first appearance as *Homo sapiens*, or modern man, with the beginning of a cerebrum, some fifty thousand years ago. Biologically, we are the same people as those prehistoric ancestors; we have the same basic nervous systems and the same pain defenses they possessed against the perils they faced—attack from animals and other humans, injury from accidents. These pain defenses are in the spinal cord and the thalamus.

Our prehistoric ancestors rarely lived long enough to suffer the major illnesses we now face, the diseases of long and comfortable life: cancer, heart attack, stroke. And in those rough days of survival of the fittest, children with diabetes, weak hearts, or the aftereffects of measles, did not survive. Man's biologic evolution stopped thousands of years before he learned to prolong his life through medicine.

While it took millions of years for man to develop biologically, his recorded history is only a few thousand years old, and his science and medicine younger even than that. In fact, it is only in the past century that most men and women have lived long enough to suffer these diseases of middle and old age.

Man's pain defense mechanisms may have been "set" in his spinal cord and thalamus before he developed his modern, thinking, cerebral cortex. As Dr. Edward Perl, a University of

North Carolina physiologist, put it in a recent essay on pain sensation: "It can be argued that the system for nociception [pain perception] evolved long before major threats to the organism were related to processes of development and aging."

So pain, a useful warning in some cases, is no warning in others. In the words of one pain researcher, it is "a senseless element of life . . . an obstacle and a threat." Pain, in addition to being a *symptom* of disease, can also *be* a disease.

Injury to nerve fibers, resulting either from accident or from nerve disease, can produce the most terrible of pains. Millions suffer the pains of arthritis. Cancer in its last stages is extremely painful. These persistent, terrible, disabling pains are among medical science's most difficult and frustrating problems. Doctors call such pain *chronic* (always) and *intractable* (untreatable).

Then there are the strange kinds of pain for which no cause at all can be found, just as no cause can be found for the opposite problem, inability to feel pain. Long after an injury has healed and damaged nerve fibers have grown back to normalcy, sufferers from spontaneous pain experience severe and unexplained tortures. A gentle touch, a breeze, a slight scratch from a thorn can trigger the most terrible of pains, lasting for days, weeks, and months. No one knows why.

Even stranger is the phenomenon called phantom limb pain, which sometimes follows amputation of a hand, foot, arm, or leg. Years after the amputation, the patient may "feel" terrible burning, cramping, or stabbing pains in the limb that is no longer there.

Phantom limb pain occurs even though the stump has healed. It is more common in patients who felt pain in the limb for some time before amputation than in those who lost a limb suddenly because of an accident. This suggests that the brain's "memory" of pain may be a cause.

In addition to the useless tortures caused by these kinds of pain, one's health is damaged by chronic pain. Constant suffering is a disease. It can disable and destroy an individual and can contribute to high blood pressure, heart disease, and emotional and psychiatric disorders.

A world without pain is impossible, but one in which pain can be controlled and unnecessary pain is eliminated is possible. It is to achieve such a world that researchers continue to study the bewildering puzzle of pain.

One part of that puzzle is the difference in the way different individuals react to pain.

Chapter 3

Why It Hurts Me More
Than It Hurts You

Long before the days of Muhammad Ali and other black champions there used to be a racist "theory" about prize-fighters' pain. Many white fans believed that all blacks were insensitive to pain in the head, but exceptionally sensitive to the pain of body blows.

In those days, during matches between "white hopes" and black champions, racist shouts would pour down from all sides of the arena, advising the white fighter: "Don't hit the nigger in the head, ye'll break yer hand! Hit him in the guts where he can't take it.!"

It was probably Joe Louis who effectively demolished this "theory" of racial pain differences when he beat Max Schmeling and other whites. Today's fans no longer admonish white fighters to aim for blacks' midsections and avoid their heads. Nor would any white fighter heed such silly advice. It is now commonly known that the supply of nerve fibers to head, abdomen, or any other part of the body does not vary from one individual to another and certainly not among racial or ethnic groups. Individuals do not differ significantly in their *sensitivity* to pain sensation.

Individuals *do* differ in their *reactions* to pain sensation, however, and it is widely believed that they have different "pain thresholds." Some are said to have a high threshold —that is, they feel pain only after considerable injury and tissue damage. Others are said to have a low threshold—they react instantly to the slightest sensation of discomfort.

A classic example of a very low threshold is the fairy tale about the princess and the pea. She was so sensitive that she could feel the pea through forty mattresses. Undoubtedly, her sensitivity was related to her being a princess: royalty and upper-class people have always been described in literature as more "sensitive" than ordinary people.

There are differences in the way individuals perceive and react to pain. There are also differences in the way a particular person will perceive pain at one time and the way he or she will perceive it at another time.

How a particular person receives and perceives the pain message—how he reacts to it, tolerates, and deals with it—is determined by his brain, and in particular by the cerebral cortex. Every cortex is unique because every human being is unique. Different human beings have had different growing-up experiences, and are therefore subject to different family and cultural influences. The cerebral cortex not only distinguishes man from other animals, but also distinguishes human beings from each other. No two human personalities are the same—although identical twins do come close.

Because each of us is different, what is a clout to one man can be a caress to another man—and can be either or neither to a woman. What hurts me may not hurt you, and it may not hurt me either the next time.

Does this mean that the racists are right and one ethnic group can withstand pain better than another? Or that one group can withstand it better in different parts of the anatomy?

No, but it does mean that we react and respond to the same pain in different ways because of the way we've been raised.

Let's take an important discriminated-against "minority" —women.

In our culture, that of the Western, primarily Christian countries, childbirth is supposed to be painful, and women are expected to suffer. They are expected to complain about the pain of labor. The Bible even states that this suffering is God's will. God tells Eve, "In sorrow thou shalt bring forth children" (Genesis 3:16). Women do feel pain during labor. Most mothers are given an anesthetic in order to make them more comfortable and also to make the doctors' and nurses' jobs easier. Yet anesthetics can be a serious threat to the newborn baby's health, and can even contribute to possible mental defects.

In some societies childbirth is *not* regarded as painful. Girls are brought up to consider giving birth a natural, painless, joyous occasion, and as women they do not appear to feel any pain at all during labor. Many young women in our culture these days are attempting—successfully—to give birth without anesthesia. This is called natural childbirth, and a growing number of doctors approve of it, except when there are medical complications.

An extreme example of the power of the culture to influence pain is couvade, a practice common among ancient European tribes and still found today in parts of Asia, Africa, and South America. In couvade (from the French word for "hatching") the woman suffers no pain in childbirth but the man does! If the man does not suffer properly, it is assumed he is not the father of the baby.

The woman shows no discomfort right up to the time of labor. At that time she stops whatever she is doing, usually working in the fields, has her baby, and then returns to her work. The man has meanwhile taken to his bed, where he groans in agony. In a particularly difficult case he may stay in bed for a day or so.

Does this mean that women in our culture really do *not* feel pain during childbirth, and are just looking for sympathy? No, because they really do hurt. Nor does it mean that some women bear the pain "better" than others. It does mean that the *way* in which the brain reacts to the pain signal is of greater importance than the sensation at the location where the tissue is actually tearing or stretching, and the brain's reactions are always strongly influenced by the culture and the way one is reared. It is in the brain that pain is felt. Most important analgesics—pain-killing drugs—work on the brain, or the pathways to it, not on the hurt tissue.

Thus, there are differences in the way different groups perceive pain, despite the fact that we all have the same pain machinery. Most little boys in our culture are raised to bear pain, and not to cry—and most little girls are *expected* to cry. And so males appear to be less sensitive to pain. All this is changing, of course, and we will say more about sex differences and pain in Chapter 12.

There are other group differences. Some years ago Dr. Mark Zborowski, a social scientist, studied Jewish, Anglo-Saxon, Irish, and Italian patients in a Veterans Administration hospital in New York City. He found interesting differences in the way each of these four groups of patients—all male, of course—reacted to the same pain.

In general, the Jews and Italians complained loudly, bitterly, and with great emotion at their pain. Most of the Anglo-Saxon patients gritted their teeth and tried to cause as little "trouble" as possible, and the tendency among the Irish patients was to suffer in silence.

The Jews and Italians, Dr. Zborowski found, saw no reason to keep their suffering to themselves. Why not complain? The Anglo-Saxons were anxious to do what they thought was "proper." The Irish believed their masculinity required them to shut up and bear their agony. The men in each of these four groups "felt" pain in accordance with the ways they were raised, in accordance with their cultural backgrounds.

There were other differences. Although the Jews and Italians appeared to react in the same way, the Jews were concerned about what the symptoms *meant*—as were the Anglo-Saxons. Both groups of patients speculated about the significance of the symptoms and would not accept analgesic drugs until they had had an explanation, a diagnosis of their pain. Did the pain mean a worsening of the disease? The Italians, however, cared only for relief from the pain and welcomed analgesics. The Irish did not even attempt to evaluate the pain, but just accepted it or tried to say it didn't really hurt too much.

The doctors also played a role. They acted as if certain pain behavior was "correct," and other behavior was "incorrect." The Jewish and Italian reactions were dismissed as "over-exaggerated, hysterical." The Anglo-Saxon reactions were considered "correct;" the Irish, "manly." Such prejudice on the part of a doctor interferes with proper treatment. It leads the doctor to ignore one patient's complaint as "hysterical,"in favor of another patient's "correct" reaction.

Other forces operate on the brain's capacity for pain perception. There are important individual differences as well as cultural. Even though we may be members of the same culture, each of us is unique. In a study at Harvard Medical School in the sixties, Dr. Asenath Petrie found that all people, regardless of culture, seem to fall into three pain categories.

She became interested in this when she observed that different hospital patients seemed to react differently to the same kind of pain. These differences seemed to have nothing to do with their backgrounds. Factors such as culture, "willpower," and sex did not seem to explain sufficiently why one patient bore pain without much reaction while another complained bitterly. Dr. Petrie also found that nurses and doctors had long noted that some patients needed more analgesic drugs after surgery than others did.

Dr. Petrie performed pain sensation experiments in the laboratory, using healthy volunteers, and found that the people she studied perceived and reacted to pain signals in one of three different ways.

One group apparently had what she called reducer personalities, and she quite naturally labeled them "reducers."
These individuals minimized and played down, or reduced,
the sensations they received in the brain. They could bear
greater amounts of pain, and they had what might be
(incorrectly) called high pain thresholds.

At the other extreme were those she described as "augmentors," those who augmented, or magnified, the sensations they received. These people had personalities that
seemed to make more of pain and of other sensations than did
the others. They reacted more to pain, and they reacted more
quickly.

A third group reacted moderately, and she called them
"moderators." They neither minimized nor magnified their
pain signals.

The differences between reducers, augmentors, and
moderators were differences in the way in which their brains
perceived pain and other sensations. Dr. Petrie suggested that
these were three different types of personalities. The personality characteristic that influences the ways in which one
responds to pain and other sensations, she said, cannot be
explained.

Dr. Petrie seemed to find the reducers the most interesting
of the three. Although these people seemed to bear pain
better, she found that this was not necessarily an advantage.
Reducers, she said, have a need for more sensation than do
other types of personalities. It is as if their brains screen out
much sensation, and so therefore sensation must be strong,
even excessive, to "get through" to the brain. But the personality needs a certain minimum level of sensation if it is to
remain healthy. Human and animal babies will not develop,
will sicken and suffer mental retardation, if they are deprived
of sensation—noise, light, touch, pain.

Too much sound, too much light, too much noise, too much
pain are damaging to mental and physical health. But the lack of
these stimuli can also be a form of torture. Prisoners are put in

solitary confinement for just this reason; the lack of sensation experienced there is as effective a form of torture as is physical pain.

When she studied teen-age prisoners in a Massachusetts jail, Dr. Petrie found that some youngsters put into solitary confinement inflicted pain on themselves. These reducers burned themselves with cigarettes and cut themselves with sharp metal in order to relieve the unbearable lack of sensation. Pain sensation was better than no sensation at all. One told her, "I'd rather be hit in the head with a hammer than locked up in isolation."

Reducers need more sensation than others. It is as if the brain were a television set, and they have their volume turned down too low. Augmentors may be said to have the volume turned up too high, moderators to have it set just right.

Extreme reducers, says Dr. Petrie, may need sensation so badly that they become aggressive and overactive, and perhaps these are the youngsters who become delinquents and later criminals. Since they do not feel pain as keenly as the rest of us, they become sadistic—indifferent to pain—as far as others are concerned.

Some pain may be an essential part of life. "Pain is life," wrote the British essayist Charles Lamb, "the sharper the more evidence of life."

Dr. Petrie's work has been criticized by other pain researchers on the ground that it is based on a small number of individuals and that much of the information on which she bases her theory is what scientists call anecdotal—bits and snippets of data that have not been carefully controlled and studied. But her theory is nevertheless a fascinating and potentially useful way of looking at pain. Even her critics say that her ideas may lead to important new findings about how personality affects reactions to pain.

One of these critics is Dr. B. Berthold Wolff of New York University Medical Center, himself an eminent pain researcher. Dr. Wolff has pioneered in measuring pain responses in patients rather than in healthy volunteers. It is his (and others') opinion that pain inflicted in the laboratory is very different from the pain one feels when he or she is actually sick, and Dr. Wolff believes that it is the latter that should be studied, although he also feels that much can be learned from laboratory experiments on healthy people.

In an experiment with sixty men and women suffering from chronic arthritis, Dr. Wolff discovered a special personality trait in some (but not all) patients. He calls this the pain endurance factor. It may explain why some people can stand pain more easily than others, and therefore need less analgesia or anesthesia, complain less, and are affected less by suffering. If the existence of such a factor is proved and scientists learn to detect its presence, physicians will be able to determine in advance precisely how much anesthesia or analgesia a particular patient will require for a particular medical or surgical procedure. Many patients now receive more of these drugs than is good for them because physicians want to make sure they do not feel pain. These are powerful drugs, some are habit-forming, and it is best to take as little as possible.

Dr. Wolff's pain endurance factor received scientific support in May, 1974, with the publication in *Science* magazine of a study of pain and personality in eighty-one men and thirty-eight women hospital patients. These patients were being treated at a Veterans Administration hospital clinic for chronic pain. The researchers found three personality factors influencing the intensity of pain: the extent to which the person felt sorry for himself or herself, the patient's understanding of the pain, and Dr. Wolff's pain endurance factor.

Our mood at the moment and the cause we see behind the pain influence our reactions to pain. We do not always feel it in the same way or to the same degree.

A banged knee doesn't hurt while skiing; a wrenched muscle is ignored during an exciting tennis match. But afterward, when the distraction of the sport is no longer present, we feel our aches and bruises keenly. Just as a busy mother tunes out her pestering child, the brain seems to say to the hurt: "Don't bother me now; I'm busy. I'll listen to you later." And later it does.

Other emotional states also influence pain perception. We hurt more when we are tired or fearful or anxious. We hurt less when we are feeling good or when we connect the pain with a good thing.

Breaking a leg is a very painful experience. For one deliberately to break one's own leg—coolly, carefully—is a very difficult thing unless one has a reason so strong it overrides the pain. If one has such a reason, the brain has to literally tune out the hurt.

Thirty-six Georgia convicts in Rock Quarry State Prison had a good reason in July, 1956. They were forced to work many hours in the hot sun, breaking stones and loading heavy wheelbarrows. No one paid any attention to their complaints. The work became torture, and the men felt they had to protest their torture in some dramatic way.

All thirty-six broke their legs with their ten-pound sledge hammers. "The men," said Georgia Director of Corrections Jack Forrester, "had placed rocks under their heels and knees during a rest period and had started whacking away with sledges used for crushing rock. There were no screams."

More than ten years before these prisoners broke their own legs, some American soldiers fighting on Anzio beachhead in Italy, in World War II, gave an even more dramatic example of how the emotions of the moment and the meaning of the pain can influence sensation. When these soldiers were wounded in battle, they showed no sign of suffering. As they were carried off to evacuation boats, only one out of three complained seriously enough to require pain-killing drugs. Most of them denied having pain, or said it wasn't bad enough for drugs. Yet they had very bad wounds.

These same soldiers complained loudly and bitterly when a nurse or doctor pricked them a little too hard with hypodermic needles!

And years later the doctor reporting these reactions asked civilians who had surgical wounds similar to the battle wounds of the soldiers if they wanted pain-killing drugs. Most of them said they did.

The doctor concluded that the pain felt was not just a simple direct sensation resulting from the wound, but was strongly influenced by other factors operating in the person's brain: how the mind evaluated the wound. The soldiers knew in advance that the wounded would be evacuated. They saw the wounds with relief, as evidence that they had survived the war and were now out of it. The clumsy needle punctures were seen as just that and were resented because they were unnecessary. And to the civilians, there was nothing to be thankful for in having to undergo surgery.

Couples locked in the passion and pleasure of sexual intercourse sometimes inflict little wounds on each other—bites, scratches, bruises. These are never noticed until much later. But similar minor pain sensations are intolerable when they are caused by nonpleasurable actions at a time when one is depressed, tired, and worried.

It would seem that pain is in the mind of the sufferer, rather than in his or her injured organ. And there is a tendency for people to assume that when something is described as "being in the mind," it's the same as saying that it doesn't really exist. This is a mistake.

Pain is controlled and perceived in the mind. But it's real all the same. Whether it's the pain of the long-suffering Anglo-Saxon patient or the vocal Jewish patient, of the man who bears his pain without complaining or the woman who screams in childbirth, of the reducer or the augmentor, of the soldier with the wound that doesn't hurt or the soldier who complains of the needle—all pain is real. But just as all of us have different brains, all of us perceive it differently.

Chapter 4

Getting Help

Taking your pain to the doctor is like describing the Mona Lisa to a blind man in a language neither of you understands.

You find it hard to put a description of your pain into words; he finds it hard to understand and interpret your pain because he doesn't know precisely what your words mean to you.

Being human, he is full of prejudices. His job is to relieve the pain and cure its cause. He may resent his frustration if he is unsuccessful in helping you. Maybe it's your fault! he thinks.

As a result of this attitude, many patients have been badly treated by doctors who dismiss their pain as "imaginary" and send them to psychiatrists. Or who say with ill-concealed contempt, "You must have a low threshold." But if you feel it, it is *not* imaginary. It's real to you. Whatever in the world "threshold" means, the doctor certainly doesn't know because no one knows. Your perception of pain sensations is known only to you.

Most doctors, of course, are truly concerned about their patients' pain and try to interpret it correctly and treat it successfully, remembering always that most pain is a symptom, not a disease. A doctor, confronted with a complaint of pain, is like a detective faced with a clue. How can this bit of information determine and track down the guilty criminal?

This is the way one textbook on medicine describes this problem: "Pain is a personal experience, and communication about it depends upon the experience and vocabulary of the sufferer, just as its interpretation depends upon the experience and bias of the listener."

But there are some general rules of evidence. By getting the patient's answers to questions—Where does it hurt? How long has it hurt? Describe the pain. Under what circumstances did it start? When does it hurt most? Does it change when you move? Does it wake you up at night?—the doctor can often narrow down the possibilities. Physical examination plus such common diagnostic tests as X rays or blood tests can refine the medical detective work even further. This is the case with simple (but very intense) pains that have clear causes: fractures, wounds, ulcers, appendicitis, kidney stones.

But some pains are complicated. Some are so puzzling they are medical whodunits that challenge the doctor's imagination and skill and require him to be a diagnostic Sherlock Holmes.

In some cases the patient is the only source of clues, and there is nothing else to rely on. Such is the case when there is some problem with the hinge of the jaw, a condition most often taken to dentists rather than to physicians. In this disease, the patient's description of how he hurts and where he hurts is the only information available. An X ray usually shows nothing; even if it does show damage to the hinge, no one knows how much damage causes how much pain. So the patient's report in his own words of how much he hurts is the only evidence on which the dentist or physician can base a diagnosis.

On the other hand, the patient's complaints of pain may be as misleading as the phony clues scattered by a tricky burglar. In the strange, inexplicable, and by no means uncommon phenomenon of *referred* pain, the pain is referred from the diseased organ to another part of the body. What hurts is not what is damaged but something else. If pain is an alarm signal, then referred pain is what happens when a burglar breaks into a house in Detroit and the alarm bell goes off in St. Louis.

Take the case of a twenty-year-old English printer who had a bad toothache. His case was so interesting it was written up in a British dental journal, for what turned out in the end to be a toothache started out as a chest pain. The printer described it as "a gripping feeling across the lower part of the ribs—just above the stomach." It spread to his jaw. This pain went on for about three weeks, while the printer took all sorts of medicine for heartburn and indigestion. Fortunately, he was too young a man to think of heart pain and to worry about that!

Quite by accident he noticed that if he pressed his tongue against one of his teeth, the pain went away temporarily. This relief followed the tongue pressure so consistently that it occurred to him that his tooth might be the problem rather than his chest or abdomen. So he went to a dentist, who found that he had an abscess in the root canal of his tooth. When this was treated, the pain went away.

There seems to be a referred-pain relationship between the heart and the teeth and jaw. A toothache that masquerades as chest pain may be upsetting, but it is certainly less dangerous than heart-attack pain disguised as a toothache. The latter might not be detected in time.

Heart attack—more accurately myocardial infarction—usually starts as a sudden and increasing chest pain accompanied by a terrible feeling of not being able to breathe. The pain may then spread to the left shoulder and jaw, and down the left arm. Myocardial infarction survivors sometimes describe the pain as running out the end of the little finger of the left hand.

At a scientific meeting considering the subject of dental pain, Dr. John I. Ingle, a dental surgeon associated with the Institute of Medicine of the National Academy of Science, recently described two cases of heart pain referred to the jaw.

"In each case," said Dr. Ingle, "no heart or chest symptoms were experienced. Nor was there the common pain referral to the left arm; only symptoms to the jaw."

The first was a man who felt sudden sharp pain in one of the molars in his left jaw while he was working in his garden. He took aspirin, felt nauseous, and vomited. The pain did not go away. The next day he saw his dentist, who could find nothing wrong with his teeth. After careful questioning, the dentist learned that while the man had no chest pain he did have some pain in his right arm—an unusual place for heart pain to be referred. The alert dentist rightly suspected that the patient had heart pain referred to his left jaw and sent him to a cardiologist—a heart specialist.

The second case ended less happily. This time the patient went to his dentist complaining of a severe stabbing pain in one of his left front teeth. He had previously had dental work near that tooth, and so he and the dentist both suspected a recurrence of the earlier problem. The dentist could find nothing wrong after testing and X-raying the tooth, but he nevertheless recommended pulling it out!

The patient refused to have the tooth out and went instead to another dentist, an endodontist who had previously given him a root-canal treatment. This dentist could not find anything wrong either, but he did see two sores on the man's gum. They looked like sores of a common mouth virus (herpes simplex) which sometimes does painful damage to the nerve cells. So he sent the man to a neurologist—a nerve disease specialist. The man refused to go. Six months later he suffered a massive heart attack; a year after that he died of what may have been his third heart attack.

The problem of pain referred from an injured or diseased organ to another part of the body is a very puzzling one for doctors trying to detect the cause of the pain. No one knows exactly how pain is referred, but it is believed the phenomenon is a result of nerve fibers from certain organs that enter the main "cable" of the spinal cord close to or at the same point as pain nerve fibers from other parts of the body. There is a sort of overlap, as if two long-distance telephone wires were crossed, and one hears someone else's conversation mixed in with one's own. You're *talking* to someone in Los Angeles, but you find yourself *listening* to someone in Houston.

The referral problem is especially confusing because most of the viscera—the inner organs of the body, such as the heart, lungs, stomach, intestines, and liver—do not have as clearly defined pain nerve fibers as do the arms and legs, muscles, and outer parts of the body, especially the skin. The viscera are on a somewhat different pain "network." Possibly because of the early development of pain as a "primitive" protective mechanism against *outside* danger or attack, the machinery for perceiving and identifying pain from *inner* organs is not as precise. This may be an additional explanation for the lack of pain from the dangerous, degenerative diseases of internal organs.

As the nerves from inner organs enter the spinal cord, they sometimes converge in the same cells as those from various sections of the outer part of the body and the skin. (See Figure 1.) Nerves from the heart and its arteries converge in the cord with nerves that carry pain from the chest, shoulder, and arm. So pain caused by narrowing of the small blood vessels carrying blood to the heart muscle—a symptom of myocardial infarction—is felt *not* as heart pain but as a general pain across the chest, arm, and jaw. It is referred to these parts of the body from the heart.

Pain referral is very puzzling for dentists because the jaw and face seem to be so often involved, although not always as dramatically as in cases of heart pain referral. Pain is referred from one tooth to another, from one part of the jaw to another, from the head or ear or eye to teeth, and vice versa. In Chapter 10 we will take up the problem of tooth pain in more detail.

The list of possible pain referrals, especially from organs deep within the body to places the patient can easily recognize as on the surface of the body, is endless. Pain from the esophagus is referred to the chest. Pain from a stomach or duodenal ulcer can be referred to just above the navel. Pain in the genital tract can be felt up high in the groin; and pain in the testicle, in the lower abdomen. Pain in the urethra is often felt as pain at the tip of the penis; pain from a kidney stone can be felt in the upper back or low in the groin.

If you gulp down an extra-large chunk of ice cream, you'll feel a sudden blinding headache all across the front of your skull, just behind your eyes. This is a common (if relatively harmless) kind of referred pain. It's caused by the vagus nerve in the stomach sending sudden massive cold signals up to the brain. The vagus nerve converges with the trigeminal nerve, which comes from the face, forehead, and jaw. So the sudden chill in your stomach is perceived as a pain in your head.

What should the physician do when a patient complains of pain that may be referred or may have no clear-cut cause? Referred pain is not as much of a problem as it sounds if the physician (or the dentist) is alert to the possibility of referral. One rule of thumb is that pain is almost never referred across

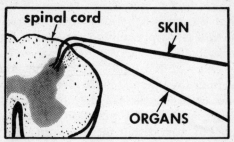

Figure 1. A possible explanation of referred pain. Sensory fibers carrying sensation messages from inner organs (heart, for example) converge with those carrying such messages from outer parts of the body and the skin as both enter the spinal cord. Pain in these organs may therefore be perceived as coming from the other parts of the body, as heart pain is often perceived as coming from the chest, arm, shoulder, or jaw.

the midline—from one side of the body to another. It's unlikely (but not impossible) that pain in the right jaw, for example, will be a symptom of heart trouble.

A good and conscientious doctor will take a detailed history of the pain, which means he will listen carefully to the patient's complaint and not dismiss it—or even seem to dismiss it—as minor or imaginary or "emotional." Dr. Berthhold Wolff puts it this way:

> I accept the patient's subjective verbal interpretation provided he mentions a part of his body. It is very hard, perhaps impossible in the ordinary practice of medicine, to detect a "malingerer"—one who complains falsely. Just because I cannot find the physical cause of the pain does not mean it is not there.

Dr. Wolff thinks that all pain falls into three categories. The most common kind, mild pain, does not interfere with the patient's ability to work or function, nor does it change his behavior. These are the "normal" pains we suffer in daily life. Such pain is the easiest for the doctor to treat, either by treating the illness, by prescribing analgesics of one kind or another, or by both.

The most severe kind of pain—the kind that is chronic and totally consumes the patient, so that he or she can think of nothing else and is in constant torment—is not, says Dr. Wolff, the biggest problem for the doctor. This kind of pain can be treated only by drastic measures, and the doctor has little choice but to use emergency procedures.

The hardest kind of pain to treat, says Dr. Wolff, is the moderately severe pain that often interferes with the patient's life. It can be treated, but the treatment may be as much of a problem as the pain itself. Such pain can result from nerve damage, from persistent headaches, or from various kinds of bone and muscle problems.

Some of these pains can be treated by psychological methods. This is because the mind—the cerebral cortex —plays so important a role in pain perception. In fact, more and more pain researchers are coming to the conclusion that all pain is a psychological event.

"Psychological" does not mean imaginary or caused by psychiatric problems, however. It means *something that happens as a result of brain activity.*

Chapter 5

You've Got to BELIEVE!

Just because something happens in the cerebral cortex doesn't mean we can think it away. If we are normal, we can no more "forget" who we are, our telephone number, our family, a mother's voice, than we can "forget" what makes us hungry or what turns us on sexually—or pain. We are what our life and experience have made us.

Nothing about pain is simple. The power of the conscious mind to control pain, or at least to make it bearable, is not simple either. The sudden savage onslaught of heart-attack pain comes with too much of a rush, rises too fast to intensity, for the mind to get it under control. Thought is relatively slow, compared to other brain processes.

But when pain is slow, or when it can be anticipated, the cerebral cortex may have time to marshal its forces of memory and consciousness, and thereby keep it under control. There are times—as with the soldiers on Anzio beachhead, who "knew" in advance that if they were wounded they'd be out of the war—when the cortex can be "prepared."

Anticipation of pain can be a time of torment for anxious people. But since men and women are blessed with an elaborate, sophisticated cerebral cortex capable of rational, thoughtful analysis, let us assume the best and consider ourselves intelligent, well-balanced individuals with the best brains available.

The power of the cortex is enormous, and it can be used for irrational and mystical ends as well as rational and scientific ones. A strongly held belief—it usually has to be religious to be strong enough—can triumph over pain nerve fibers, and can even prevent injury to tissues.

Such is the case, *most of the time*, with the fire walkers of India. These fire walkers walk barefoot on hot coals to demonstrate both their belief in Kali—the Hindu goddess representing both life and death, the unity of creation and destruction—and their confidence that she will protect them. It is not a ritual of endurance or of "manly" indifference to pain.

The object of the fire walking is not to overcome pain but to *escape* it, not to bear injury but *to be uninjured*. The fire walkers and the believers who come to observe them believe that pain or damage to the skin of the feet is evidence of failure. This failure may be due either to abandonment by the goddess Kali, who will no longer protect her followers, or to some violation of ritual by the fire walkers themselves.

Do these fire walkers really suffer no pain? Do they suffer no tissue damage to the soles of their feet? James Freeman, an anthropologist with many years of experience studying religion and culture in the Indian state of Orissa, has personally observed about twenty-five people walk over hot coals. Not all of them walked successfully, but those who did seemed to suffer neither pain nor damage to the skin of their feet.

"I am not a medical doctor," Professor Freeman told me, "and my judgments about tissue damage are not those of an expert. One man who walked successfully said he sometimes gets small blisters—so small that they are neither readily noticeable to others nor annoying or painful to him.

"Those who are burned had large blisters covering most of the foot, were in considerable pain, and limped noticeably for days."

Clearly, not all fire walkers are successful. "I have twice visited one community," said Professor Freeman, "in which the main attraction involves walking three times over a path of coals 180 feet long. In 1963 I saw three devotees attempt this ordeal. Two of them made the full run. The third stopped after 120 feet, even though the kalasi, the semipriestly representatives of Kali, threatened him with divine punishment. I was not able to see their feet, but a reliable informant told me that it is not uncommon for fire walkers to suffer extensive tissue damage."

Professor Freeman speculates about all the possible explanations for those who do not suffer pain or burns. Are the soles of their feet tougher? Is the fire perhaps not as hot as it appears to be? ("I stood as close as I could, two or three feet away," he says, "and I found it much too painful to get any closer.") Is there some trick in the way fire walkers place their feet? Is the sacred water they dip their feet into at the beginning of the run in some way protective? Do the fire walkers hypnotize themselves?

Professor Freeman, a good scientist, is careful to say that he has no evidence to prove or disprove any of these or other explanations. But he believes that the real explanation is probably psychological; that the successful fire walkers, because of the strength of their belief in Kali and in their own purity, are able to control (through their cerebral cortex?) their reactions to the fire, including the reactions of the tissues of their feet.

In the spring of 1972 Professor Freeman witnessed a spectacular failure at a village in which ten of fifteen experienced fire walkers, including a kalasi, were badly burned. The villagers, believing that Kali had deserted them, were thrown into a state of panic and confusion. One of the five successful walkers was a village "magician" who had not prepared spiritually for the ceremony in the usual fashion, who had quarreled with a leading kalasi (the one who was later burned!), and who had boasted that he could walk safely on the fire despite his lack of proper preparation.

What caused the failure? Professor Freeman believes that the magician's quarreling and boastful challenge, plus the delay it caused in the start of the ceremony, upset and unnerved the fire walkers. "They became disconcerted and flustered by the magician's antics," he reasons. "They lost the psychological concentration they needed to control their reactions."

As for the five who were successful, they had clearly *not* lost their psychological state of preparedness. And as for the "nonbelieving" magician, his belief in his own magic was apparently strong enough to protect him.

In short, with some kinds of pain perception, it may be enough to *believe* one will be unhurt, provided one believes it strongly.

It may also be enough to *understand*. In our presumably rational culture where no one in his right mind would attempt to walk on fire, we must undergo other, unfortunately necessary, tortures in certain forms of medical treatment. A series of fascinating experiments is proving that the power of the mind to *understand* and to *anticipate* such necessary pain and discomfort can diminish it. Where no analgesia is possible, knowledge may be the essential pain-killer.

These experiments on the effect of providing prior information have been and are still being conducted by Dr. Jean E. Johnson of the Center for Health Research of the Wayne State University College of Nursing in Michigan. Dr. Johnson's work has great value for nurses and others who are responsible for helping people bear discomfort and pain.

She has been experimenting with that necessary but frightening form of medical torture known as endoscopy, in which a tube is put down a patient's throat into the stomach. This is done so that the doctor can both look at and take pictures of the upper gastrointestinal tract. It is an important diagnostic procedure when a patient has a recurrent and apparently untreatable pain or obstruction in the tract, and is often necessary in order to see just exactly what the problem may be so that it can be treated.

An endoscopic examination may not sound as bad as walking barefoot on hot coals, but it is not much better. Here is what happens:

1. The throat is swabbed with a local anesthetic, something like novocaine, to reduce sensation,

2. A vein in the arm or wrist is punctured for injection of a steady flow of tranquilizer,

3. A flexible tube about as thick as a thumb is passed down through the mouth and throat into the stomach. It is kept there from fifteen to thirty minutes while the doctor looks and takes pictures through it. Then it is removed.

This examination can be done safely and successfully only if the patient is *not* anesthetized and is able to follow certain instructions. The patient has to breathe through the mouth, make swallowing motions as the tube moves down, and change position during the examination at the request of the doctor.

"How," asks Dr. Johnson, "can we prepare a person to make him or her react less to fearful emotions, and more to instructions, during the endoscopic examination?" In order to help answer that question, she and her associates conducted experiments on forty-eight endoscopy patients at the University of Wisconsin Medical Center.

All forty-eight were visited by a physician the day before the examination and were given the information endoscopy patients ordinarily received. They were told they would receive sedatives in their rooms to calm them down. They were told where the examinations would be done; that their throats would be painted to make them numb; that they would receive injections of a tranquilizer drug in an arm vein, which would make them drowsy but allow them to stay awake; that the tube would be as thick as a thumb; and that other patients had had the examination and did not find it difficult.

Ten of the patients received only this standard preparation and no more information. They were what scientists call controls, that is, "normal" subjects against whose performance the other, experimental subjects' performance would be measured. This is classic experimental procedure. Without controls no experiment is valid.

A second group of fourteen experimental patients received special instructions on what the procedure was all about and *how to behave* during it. These patients were told to breathe rapidly through the mouth and to pant during the throat painting in order to reduce gagging. And they were told how to act while the tube was going down: to make swallowing motions with the mouth open and the chin down.

These patients were given tape recordings of this information, and were encouraged to practice while the tape was played. They were given additional practice sessions after the tape was over.

A third group of thirteen experimental patients received information in advance about what *sensations* to expect. They received a tape of this information plus a booklet of eleven photographs illustrating different stages of the endoscopy. One photograph, for example, showed a patient's face and position while his throat was being painted. The tape described exactly what the patient could expect to see, feel, taste, and hear.

A fourth group of eleven experimental patients received not only instructions about how to *behave* but also information about the sensations they would feel.

The patients who received information only about the sensations they would feel—who were carefully prepared in terms of their own fears—did very much better than the control group who received only the standard information; they did better than the patients who received instructions as to how to behave; and, in most cases, did even better than the patients who received both kinds of information. The third group needed less of the tranquilizer; their heart rates were more stable, indicating less fear; and it took less time to pass the tube into their stomachs.

Ninety percent of the patients who received no special information gagged. More than 57 percent of the patients receiving instructions on how to behave gagged. Only 46 percent of those who were told what sensations to expect gagged.

"Preparatory instructions," Dr. Johnson concludes, "can reduce distress." Reactions to threatening events, she adds, can be reduced if the patient is accurately informed of what to expect.

The power of the mind to alter and control pain perception is established, whether the control is by *belief*, as with the fire walkers of India, by *intelligence*, as with Dr. Johnson's informed endoscopy patients, or by the use of mind-changing drugs. But pain can be neither understood nor mastered by mind alone. We must put the cerebral cortex in its proper perspective as a part of the whole complex mechanism by which pain works.

Chapter 6

What the Pain System Is

Although pain is psychological—it occurs in the mind—it is also neurological. It requires a nervous system. Some mechanism must carry the message of a stubbed toe to the cerebral cortex, which tells one: "I have stubbed my toe." Between the telephone mouthpiece in, say, California, and the telephone earpiece in, say, New York, there must be wires, relays, main trunks, and switchboards. Such is the nervous system, a structure common, in varying degrees of complexity, to all animals from the simple earthworm to the billion-celled human being at the top of the developmental ladder.

Pain is only one of the many messages carried by the nervous system. That complicated network also carries messages about the outside environment (temperature, light, sound, taste, smell), about the inner body needs (blood pressure needs, oxygen needs, food needs, water needs), and about the bewildering variety of events and relationships—physical, anatomical, physiological—without which life could not continue. The electric messages carried by the nerves and the chemical messages carried by the hormones are the basis of life itself. But we are concerned here only about that single but certainly not least important message, pain.

In a way the nervous system is very much like a telephone system. Yet we must not stress the telephone parallel too much because the nervous system is much more complex.

When we consider the brain, we will see that it is much more comparable to a computer—the fastest, most complex computer known. But still the nervous system has its "wires"—its chains of nerve cells that bundle together to form nerve fibers. It has its "relays" and "junctions" at dorsal ganglia, where the body's thirty-one pairs of pain nerve fibers, one from each side of the body, enter the "main trunk" of the spinal cord. And the nervous system has its complex "switchboard" mechanism in the thalamus—still little understood—which selects and transmits messages to the cortex, and carries messages back down the system from the cortex to various parts of the body.

This system carries two kinds of basic messages, *sensory* and *motor*, and a third, extremely sophisticated kind of message, *interneural*. Sensory messages are about sensations (heat, cold, pressure, pain) and are carried from the body to the spinal cord and brain. Motor messages are action commands from the brain and spinal cord that tell muscles and glands what to do ("Drop that hot poker!"). Interneural messages are high-level communiqués between different parts of the brain ("Why does my left foot itch?"), between the brain and the spinal cord ("Scratch that itch!") or vice versa, and between motor and sensory nerve cells ("That scratching feels good!").

The private foot soldier of this communications army is the neuron, the nerve cell. We are concerned primarily with the sensory neurons, since they carry pain (plus other) messages. But all neurons are fundamentally alike. They are cells specialized to receive and transmit electric impulses.

Neurons are strangely shaped cells; they are by far the biggest in the body—some as long as three feet! And they are the most highly specialized. A neuron looks (see Figure 2) something like a kite, with the cell body the kite itself. But it is irregularly shaped, unlike the usual triangular or four-sided shape of most kites, and it has many projections. These projections, the dendrites, are the receiving part of the

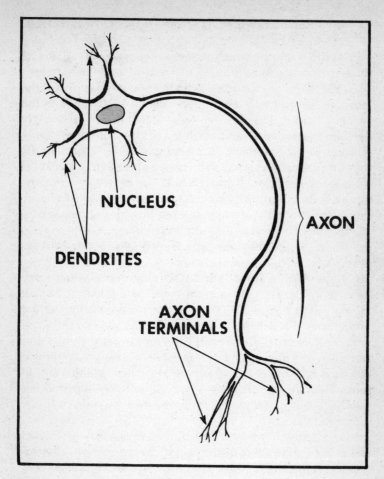

Figure 2. Diagram of a neuron.

neuron's communications system, functioning something like radio or television antennae.

A message is received at the neuron's dendrites in the form of an electric impulse, pumped down through the neuron's body to and through the "tail" of the "kite," the axon. The axon is the terminal, which passes the message along, via its clusters of tiny projections, to the next neuron's dendrites.

To pass from one neuron's axon to another's dendrites, the message has to jump a tiny gap called a synapse. It is the synapse that makes the nervous system so bewilderingly flexible. The synapse can be either a bridge facilitating transmission or a barrier inhibiting transmission. Like a traffic cop, the chemical-electric interchange at the synapse may let some messages through while it holds up others. Exactly how this is done is not really understood, but it is an extremely important process. Later we will see how the synapses play crucial roles either in letting unpleasant messages through to the brain, where they are experienced as pain, or in stopping them, so that no pain is felt.

Groups of axons are collected in wirelike nerves which carry innumerable messages simultaneously, much as the new Bell System cable carries 108,000 telephone conversations at the same time. We will try to avoid the numbers game in describing how many messages the nerves can carry, or how fast they carry the messages. But it is useful to know that in some the messages travel fast (perhaps 245 miles an hour) and in some they are slow (slower than one mile an hour). These numbers are guesstimates; different neuroanatomists give different rates.

We do have to understand that the electric messages carried along the nerves move at spectacular speeds with astronomical complexity. Before Hank Aaron's ash-wood bat connected with that pitched ball in Cincinnati in April, 1974, for home run number 714, how fast did the message move from his eyes up his spinal cord to his brain, down his spinal cord again to his arm, shoulder, feet, leg, wrist, and finger muscles? How many synapses contributed their bit? How many motor and sensory neurons? How many interneurons?

We don't know.

When we take a closer look at how neurons transmit the tiny

electric signals we call nerve impulses, we see that neurons are not at all like wires—which lie passively as *conductors* of electricity. Neurons are living cells, and they participate *actively* in the electrical transmission of nerve messages.

In passing a message it has received from its dendrites to its axon, a neuron consumes energy. Laboratory experiments have shown that the temperature of the axon increases slightly as the signal moves along, and that the neuron's output of carbon dioxide increases. Both of these are signs that the work of metabolism—which is a biologic term referring to the active processes necessary to life—is going on.

The action performed by the neuron when it is stimulated is pumping. It pumps sodium and potassium ions into and out of its cell wall. An ion is an atom or group of atoms with an electric charge. The atoms of some chemicals, including sodium and potassium, become ionized when in water. Since the human body is at least 70 percent water and contains plenty of sodium and potassium (as well as other chemicals), the conditions for producing electric charges are present.

The neuron's pumping action, which changes the chemical balance between the sodium and potassium inside and outside the neuron, gives the cell its electric charge (about seventy thousandths of a volt) and thus fires the electric impulse down the axon. The neuron then releases a chemical transmitter which carries the message to the dendrites of the next neuron, which in turn fires off an electric charge, and so on.

Through this process such diverse messages as the taste of chocolate, a message coming from the sensory neurons of the tongue, and the prick of a pin, coming from the sensory neurons of the skin, are translated into electric and chemical signals that the cerebral cortex understands as "chocolate" and "pain." Exactly *how* this is done is a mystery. Neurophysiologists will puzzle over this mystery for some time to come.

They will also puzzle over the mystery of how other neurons

carry action messages to the muscles, glands, and vital organs. The riddle of the human nervous system and its functioning is proving more difficult to unravel than the riddle of traveling to, understanding, and living in space. No communications satellite, no space control computer system, is as condensed and tightly organized as the human nervous system. The human brain, for example, weighs only about three pounds.

Sensory neurons specialize in *receiving* messages, and the different types of sensory neurons are further specialized. Some pick up only visual messages and are naturally found only in the eye. Taste, smell, and hearing neurons are found only in the tongue, nose, and ear. The neurons of touch, however, are distributed all over the skin surface, with more in some places (fingertips) than in others (the back). These neurons respond not only to touch but also to other mechanical stimuli, such as stretching, pinching, pressure, and even the movement of a single hair.

Other neurons are specialized to respond only to heat or to cold but only when the temperature falls into the normal nondamaging (that is, nonpainful) range of between approximately 54° F. and 113° F. Above and below these temperatures, there is damage to tissues, and the "pain" neurons therefore begin to fire off their electric "pain" messages.

The word "pain" is put in quotes because it is really incorrect to call these neurons pain neurons. Since pain is a cerebral, psychological concept, a neuron (which is mindless) cannot feel pain. It can only transmit messages that the brain interprets as pain. Neuroanatomists and other researchers use the rather evasive substitute word "noxious"—which means unpleasant or injurious—to describe the nature of the stimuli and of the messages these neurons and nerves respond to and transmit.

What triggers these noxious messages? How does a "pain" neuron "know" it has received a "pain" message?

In skin and muscle tissue, damage of any kind causes an immediate chemical response. The hurt cells release a family of chemicals known as polypeptides, most commonly a member of that family known as bradykinin. Bradykinin causes the tiny blood vessels to expand, and also causes the cell walls in surrounding areas to swell with fluid. These chemical and pressure changes trigger an instantaneous "pain" response from "pain" receptor neurons.

Neurons specialized to receive noxious messages are found all over the skin surface, in muscles, and in connective tissue just below the skin, but not very often in internal organs. These neurons are part of the primitive protective aspect of pain. They tell the individual when and where he or she has been burned, stabbed, struck, or otherwise injured.

"Pain" neurons are not evenly distributed on the outside of the body, which is why injuries in certain places hurt more than those in others. The eye probably has the greatest number, as anyone who has ever had a speck of dust or dirt under the eyelid knows. The eye is the most sensitive and vulnerable of the body's external organs, and this may be why this concentration of protective noxious-sensitive neurons and the protective blinking reflex evolved.

Axons in a group form nerves. "Pain" nerves are different from those that carry heat, cold, touch, and pressure messages. The "pain" nerves are thinner, and therefore transmit their messages many times more slowly than do others. The fact that "pain" nerves are the slowest plays an important role in the way we feel (and do not feel) pain.

Sensory nerves of all kinds from neighboring parts of the body meet as they approach the spinal cord and join in a dorsal root ganglion—a kind of first-stage switchboard or junction—before entering the cord itself. There are thirty-one pairs of these main nerves, half from each side of the body. There are also twelve pairs of cranial (which means skull) nerves in the head, half on each side. The cranial nerves go directly to the lower brain. The sixty-two body nerves send their various messages up the cord to the thalamus, where they too are relayed to various parts of the brain, evaluated, and acted upon. That is, decisions are made at this, the body's command post, and the resulting messages are sent down the

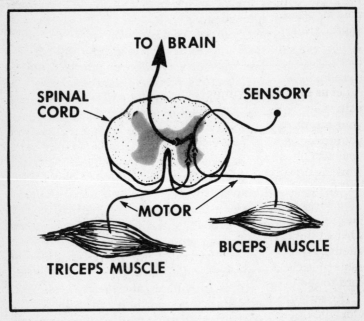

Figure 3. How the reflex arc works. A "pain" message carried by sensory fiber coming, for example, from the hand, crosses the spinal cord and triggers impulses in motor fibers going back to the muscles of that arm. These motor impulses "tell" the biceps muscle to contract and the triceps muscle to relax. These actions pull the hand away from the unpleasant sensation, all in a fraction of a second, while at the same time the sensory message is transmitted up to the spinal cord to the brain. Here the sensory message is perceived as "pain."

cord (via interneural neurons) to muscles and glands (via motor neurons).

Fast as it is, this process is not fast enough to blink an eye or pull back from the touch of a hot object. These protective reflex actions have to be done before there is time for thought. For this to happen, muscles must be given commands before central headquarters in the brain has had time to evaluate the pain message. This is accomplished by the reflex arc, a kind of short circuit in which the message from the pain fiber jumps across the spinal cord to trigger a reaction from a motor fiber. (See Figure 3.) This process is even more complicated than it sounds.

Let us say you unwittingly touch a hot cup. The protective pain reflex is to pull your arm away, a process that requires your biceps muscle, inside your upper arm, to contract. But your triceps muscle outside your arm, which works to extend your arm, must be inhibited. Otherwise the two muscles will work against each other—both will contract—and nothing will happen.

So the pain message from the sensory nerve fiber has to jump across the spinal cord and send a message via one motor fiber to the biceps ("Contract!") while it sends another via another motor fiber to the triceps ("Do nothing!"). And at the same time the sensory nerve sends a reporting message up the cord to the thalamus and the cerebral cortex.

The cortex is not necessarily a passive partner in this reflex. Our consciousness, influenced by our life experience and our memory of that experience, can play a powerful role. A good example of this has been offered by Dr. Ronald Melzack of McGill University, whose significant contribution to our understanding of pain mechanisms is described in Chapter 7.

Dr. Melzack reminds us that if we inadvertently pick up a hot object and know that it is an extremely valuable object —say a rare Wedgwood cup—our cortex tries to inhibit our reflex, which is to drop it. We will, if we know its value, juggle the cup toward a table in an attempt to save it from damage, even while we experience the pain of burning. This is an example of the conscious cerebral cortex modifying the unthinking pain reflex.

The sensory nerve fibers of the body that carry pain messages send them into the spinal cord, where they cross to the other side of the cord (from left to right, or right to left) before going up the cord into the brain. The cord, sheathed in the protective vertebrae of the spine, is connected to sensory nerve fibers from all over the body much as a great river is fed by streams and tributaries. The spinal cord travels up to the neck and skull, where it swells out, like a river entering the ocean, to become the brain. Here pain signals end, and pain is perceived.

If the spinal cord is cut and one looks at a cross section, holding it with the back part on top, one sees a perfectly symmetrical gray butterfly shape surrounded by white. (See Figure 4.) The gray "butterfly" in the center is composed primarily of neuron cell bodies; the white surrounding it is composed of the axons going up or down the cord. The upper part of each "wing" of the butterfly, just about where the antennae ought to be, is the place where the sensory nerve fibers, including those fibers that carry pain messages, enter the cord.

This part of the "butterfly" is the substantia gelatinosa, a column of small, closely packed neurons that extends the whole length of the spinal cord. The nerve fibers carrying pain messages end here. The substantia gelatinosa cells are closely connected with each other but do not send axons—that is, they do not send nerve impulses—directly to the other parts of the spinal cord or the brain. The pain and other sensory impulses are picked up by the dendrites of very large cells (neuroanatomists call them T-cells) which lie farther inside the spinal cord. These large T-cells then send the messages received through their own axons to the nerve fibers that travel up the cord to the thalamus. (More about this in Chapter 8.)

The thalamus is a large egg-shaped part of the brain which receives sensory messages from all parts of the body and relays them to the cerebral cortex. But it does more than passively pass messages along like a mailman. It reacts in an as yet little understood way. Nerve cells have the ability to excite or inhibit other nerve cells. The nerve cells of the thalamus can stir up (and be stirred up by) those of the cortex. And the nerve cells of the thalamus can also turn those of the cortex off (and be turned off by them).

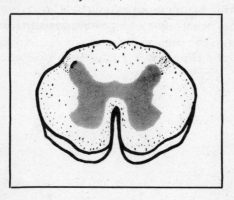

Figure 4. Cross section of the spinal cord, showing gray butterfly shape of neuron cell bodies.

The thalamus was the first part of the brain to develop; the cortex was the latest, and is the most sophisticated. The brains of animals low down on the evolutionary ladder, such as fish and birds, are all thalamus and no or very little cerebral cortex. These animals are not very bright. Those higher up, such as chimpanzees, have relatively more cortex and are more intelligent. Man, at the top of the ladder, has the largest cortex; hence his large skull and superior intelligence.

The cortex itself cannot act on pain until the thalamus relays a pain message to it. But as we have already seen, the cortex plays a major role in pain perception, as it does in all other brain activity. And even though its actions are determined by the signals coming up the spinal cord and through the thalamus, the cortex can also *control* what comes up the cord. *It can tell the thalamus what to tell it!*

The human brain is often described these days as a sort of computer. But the bewilderingly complex relationship between the cerebral cortex and the rest of the brain makes it much more sensitive and intricate a mechanism. Unlike a computer, the brain can actually determine its own input. It can "decide" what signals will be received.

This then is the basic architecture of the pain communications network. How it works is something else.

Chapter 7

How the Pain System Works

We have to begin this chapter on a discouraging note. The truth is, no one really knows just how the pain system works.

"Knowing" in the scientific sense means being able to prove, through observation and experimentation, exactly what happens and how it happens. "Proof" means tracing the pain message from the source—the painful stimulus—all the way through the nervous system, neuron by neuron, synapse by synapse, fiber by fiber, up to the brain. Scientists have charted part of the process in some cases. But in no case has a pain message been mapped past the thalamus. How and by what means such messages get to the cerebral cortex, where pain is perceived, is still a mystery.

The mechanisms by which the neurons, fibers, and ganglia transmit sensory messages to the spinal cord and across it to motor neurons—the reflex arc—are well understood. But what turns noxious sensory messages into what we call pain is only dimly guessed at. The thalamus and beyond—the complex inner workings of the brain—are largely unknown.

In laboratory experiments scientists have put a noxious stimulus at at the end of a nerve fiber and traced the electric impulse it triggers to the spinal cord and up that cable to the brain. Cats, dogs, and monkeys (as well as other animals) have had their nervous systems wired up so that noxious stimuli can be watched and measured on oscilloscopes and other instruments. We know something about what happens along the incoming lines, but not much about how the central switchboard handles and chooses among incoming calls. And we know almost nothing about the electrical and chemical processes that translate the call into a pain message.

There is an analogy in space exploration. We've sent satellites into space; we can live and work there; and we have landed on the moon. We've looked at the lunar landscape and some of the planets with television cameras and other sensory machines, and we have received from these devices data-filled messages contributing to our knowledge of our solar system. So we have a glimmering of the reality out there, as we have a glimmering of the reality inside our busy, restless brains.

But it's just a glimmer. We don't really know what the moon and the planets are like. We won't until we can live and work and study there. We know perhaps less about our own cerebral cortices and thalami, and how these play their part in the strange experience we call pain.

Yet all is not lost. Our cerebral cortices are brilliantly adapted for that highest of functions, speculating rationally and abstractly about the nature of things.

One need not know how and why a process works in order to deal with it, use it, and study it. Men knew how to sail and navigate thousands of years before they learned the physical laws governing the action of wind and water, the characteristics of airfoils and vacuums, or the forces ruling the movement of heavenly bodies. Ancient Phoenicians and Polynesians thought—with one part of their cerebrums—that gods and demons filled their sails with wind and drove their ships to safety or destruction. With another part of their brains these master navigators stored up and remembered acute observations about how to rig a sail, tack into the wind, and navigate by a star. Their ignorance of the *science* of navigation and seamanship did not keep them from crossing seas and oceans without instruments—something that we, with all our scientific knowledge, cannot do.

Ancient man knew that fermented fruits or grain produced a tasty drug that relieved pain. *We* call it alcohol, and *we* know all about the chemical process by which it is made and how it affects the cerebral cortex to kill pain. *He* did not know its chemical formula or its mechanism of action, but *he* knew how to make and use it.

Only after man had accumulated sufficient information about the world could he begin to speculate intelligently. To speculate intelligently means to think up hypotheses— intelligent guesses.

Intelligent speculation about pain had to wait for the accumulation of accurate knowledge about the anatomy and structure of the nervous system, something that began only 150 years ago. This speculation has since produced a number of hypotheses about the pain system and how it works. The most important and influential of these, the basis for many medical textbooks dealing with pain mechanisms, states that there is a "private line" for pain.

This private line is said to lead from specific neurons which receive pain stimuli, along separate nerve fibers, up a separate spinal cord "cable" to a separate, specific pain center somewhere in the brain. Many neurophysiologists accept this hypothesis for a very good reason: it is accurate and provable *as far as it goes*.

There are, as we have seen, special pain-receiving neurons in the skin which transmit their messages along special nerve fibers to a separate bundle of fibers going up the spinal cord to the thalamus. This is a different sensory system from the others that receive and transmit messages about pressure, for instance, or change of position. And the private pain line does go—together with other sensory nerve lines—to a special area in the rear of the thalamus. One could, if one wished, call this a pain center. This private line for pain sends its messages at a much slower speed than the other sensory lines. Pain messages take longer than pressure, vibration, or other touch messages, as if they were coming from a greater distance.

All of the above has been demonstrated in the laboratory by experiments. There is also some clinical evidence (meaning evidence related to the treatment of patients outside the laboratory, in real life) supporting this hypothesis. For example, if a surgeon cuts the part of the spinal cord that carries the pain fibers, and only that part, he can relieve chronic, intense pain. This surgery will not interfere with the patient's ability to feel touch or vibration sensations.

Stimulation of the slow pain fibers at the same time that the fast touch fibers are blocked by a local anesthetic causes intense pain—further evidence of a private line. And stimulating the rear part of the thalamus—the so-called pain center—also causes intense pain. Destruction of nerve fibers that feed into the thalamus from the nonpain part of the spinal cord—leaving the line open only to pain messages—causes what is called thalamic pain.

So there is indeed a private line for pain from neurons in the skin or inner organs to a special place in the brain. But this is not enough to explain all pain. There are holes in the hypothesis.

While cutting the spinal cord does relieve some types of chronic pain, this relief is usually only temporary. The pain eventually returns, sometimes even more intensely. It seems to find new pathways around the cut in the cord. Yet spinal cord fibers cannot regenerate.

The neurons in the pain center of the thalamus do respond to noxious messages. But they also respond to nonnoxious messages. So it is more than just a pain center. How does the thalamus discriminate between the two kinds of messages —pain and nonpain?

More damaging to the private-line hypothesis is the fact

that it does not explain the pain puzzles discussed in earlier chapters. A direct line from skin neurons to a pain center cannot explain why an amputee feels pain in a foot or hand that has long since been cut off. It does not explain the strange relationships or the apparent lack of any relationship between the source and the feeling (or lack of feeling) of pain: the soldiers on Anzio who did not seem to mind their bloody wounds, but who complained about the doctors' needles; the fire walkers of India who (sometimes) do not feel pain or suffer damage to their tissues; the fact that pain-killing drugs work differently with different people; the strange cases of excruciating pain caused by a light touch; the fact that one woman can have her baby without analgesia and without apparent pain, while another screams in agony if she is not put entirely to sleep.

Good as it is, the direct-private-line-for-pain hypothesis does not explain the powerful effect of the mind on pain. Something is missing.

In 1965 two scientists attempted, with a new pain hypothesis, to supply the missing elements. This was the gate control hypothesis, first published in *Science* magazine by Dr. Ronald Melzack, a psychologist at Montreal's McGill University, and Dr. Patrick Wall, then a biologist at the Massachusetts Institute of Technology, now at Oxford University. Before we examine this new hypothesis, let us back up a bit and think about hypotheses in general.

Someone once said that a hypothesis doesn't have to be *pure* or *good*; it only has to be *productive*. What's important is not whether it is right or wrong so much as what doors it opens, what new ideas it leads to.

Some examples:

From the mother hypothesis *"The world is round,"* Columbus developed the baby hypothesis "One can sail due west from Spain and reach the Indies of the East."

He had, of course, no way of knowing that his path was blocked by North and South America. So he "stumbled" on the New World and never got to the East.

Was he a failure, as he thought? Was the original hypothesis "wrong"?

Closer to our time, consider the birth control pill. Dr. John Rock, Dr. Gregory Pincus, and the rest of their team of reproductive biologists were looking, back in the 1950's, for a way to help women who could not have children. Experimenting with the female sex hormones estrogen and progesterone, they hypothesized that because these played such an important role in the reproductive cycle and especially in ovulation, they might be manipulated in such a way as to cause women who failed to ovulate to do so—to produce eggs capable of fertilization. But, in fact, the investigators "stumbled" on the opposite, a combination of estrogen and progesterone that would *keep* women from ovulating. Thus the birth control pill was born.

Were Drs. Rock and Pincus failures? Was their hypothesis "wrong"?

Such is the nature of pure science, and such is the way in which many scientific discoveries are stumbled upon. One must therefore think of an hypothesis as a candle in the dark. It may not show us what we are looking for, but it may show us what is *there*, provided that its light is bright enough and provided that we shine it in the right direction.

The community of pain researchers and doctors who treat pain has been thrown into debate by the gate control hypothesis of Drs. Melzack and Wall. This hypothesis attempts to explain all of the pain mystery, including the pain puzzles the private-line hypothesis does *not* explain. In fact gate control is the *only* pain idea that attempts to offer a single, unified, total explanation of all kinds of pain.

Dr. Melzack has modified his basic hypothesis a number of times in order to meet the criticisms of fellow scientists. Important details of his idea have yet to be proved—or disproved. Yet gate control has earned its place in the history of pain research on the basis of three giant accomplishments.

It offers the first successful explanation of the power of the mind—the cerebral cortex—over pain. This explanation has been of enormous help in understanding how pain-killing drugs work and in guiding research aimed at finding new and better analgesic drugs.

The gate control hypothesis offers plausible, if not yet provable, explanations of some of the pain puzzles already described: prolonged pain, phantom limb pain, congenital analgesia, and extreme sensitivity to ordinarily nonpainful stimuli.

But probably its most sensational accomplishment is that it is making possible the treatment of patients suffering from hitherto untreatable chronic pain. In place of the crippling and often ineffective surgical cutting of the spinal cord, there is now the new technique of electrical stimulation of nerve fibers. This form of treatment, the child of gate control thinking, has brought dramatic relief to some patients. Gate control also offers a possible explanation of how and why acupuncture may kill pain. And it seems to explain the power of psychological attitudes over pain.

The debate over gate control is roughly between researchers who cannot prove its validity by traditional experimental means and those doctors who have used it successfully to treat hopeless patients, and who couldn't care less about how or why it works. It is enough for them that treatment based on the hypothesis relieves pain.

Researchers are rightly suspicious of new scientific ideas that cannot be proved in their own laboratories. When scientists repeat experiments on which new ideas are based and obtain the same results as the original experimenter, this kind of proof is called replication. It is an important step in establishing scientific truths. If I cannot repeat your experiment myself, if it does not work for me, when I follow the same procedure, as it does for you, then your results cannot be valid. Many important details of the gate hypothesis cannot be proved; Drs. Melzack and Wall's experiments cannot always be replicated with the same results that they obtained.

Yet despite these shortcomings, the idea of a gate that controls our perception of pain messages has all the attractiveness of any imaginative new hypothesis. It answers some ancient questions and raises some new ones. It lights a candle.

Chapter 8

The Pain Gate

In the tip of each "butterfly wing" of the spinal cord (if you look at it in cross section, as in Figure 4), there is a grayish jelly. This column of jelly runs up both sides of the cord from the small of the back, where the backbone begins, to high into the neck, where the cord meets the brain.

Scientists, who like to give things Latin or Greek names, call this jelly the substantia gelatinosa, which in Latin means simply "jellylike substance." More specifically, it is a tight-packed column of neurons, and as has already been discussed in Chapter 6, these neurons (more correctly interneurons) synapse only with each other, send messages only to each other, and excite each other.

This rather closed neural world is not, however, entirely isolated. It is penetrated by dendrites from very large neurons deeper in the spinal cord, just outside the jelly. The axons of these T-cells connect with, and become part of, the main communications fiber-"cable" going up to the brain. They are important relays in the communications system.

From outside the bony spinal column, the thirty-one pairs of peripheral nerve fibers feeding in from all parts of the body on both sides deliver their sensory messages—pain, pressure, vibration, heat, cold, etc.—to the substantia gelatinosa. *It is in the substantia gelatinosa that these fibers synapse with the T-cells.*

(The twelve pairs of cranial nerves do not, of course, enter the substantia gelatinosa, but pass directly into the brain.)

The substantia gelatinosa is, then, a way station where incoming nerve fibers deliver their messages to the receiving dendrites of T-cells. T-cells *may or may not* pass these messages on up the cord to the brain, where they are received and perceived. Messages, as we know, must pass to the brain to be "real." If you do not feel a sensation, it does not exist—for you.

The cells of the substantia gelatinosa have, according to the gate control hypothesis, a powerful influence on the T-cells as they receive incoming messages. If the T-cells do not receive and transmit, the message does not go through. This is why, according to Dr. Melzack, the gray jelly in the "butterfly wing tip" is in fact the pain gate.

These close-packed neurons make their own contribution to the transmission of pain messages, even though they "talk" only to each other in what must "sound" (if neurons make any noise) like a steady buzz of chatter and conversation. Getting a pain message past them is, according to the hypothesis, a complicated matter. Sometimes they keep messages from reaching the T-cells. Sometimes they permit the messages to pass through. When the substantia gelatinosa is passive and "open," pain messages get through; when it is active and "closed," they do not.

How does this gate work? What opens it? What closes it?

The neurons in the substantia gelatinosa are turned on by messages from large nerve fibers. These are messages of pressure, vibration, touch, etc. The neurons are turned off by messages from small fibers, pain messages. When the neurons are turned on, when they are active, they send messages to the T-cells by means of dendrites embedded among them. When the neurons are turned off, they send no messages.

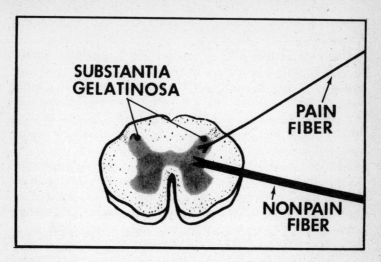

Figure 5. According to the Melzack-Wall hypothesis, there is, in the substantia gelatinosa, a pain gate that is opened by impulses from slow, thin, pain-carrying fibers, and closed by those from fast, thick fibers carrying other kinds of sensations.

The message the substantia gelatinosa send to T-cells is one of inhibition: *active* substantia gelatinosa cells mean *inactive*, nontransmitting, T-cells. And vice versa.

Turning on the substantia gelatinosa, which is what large non-pain fibers do, closes the pain gate. Turning off the substantia gelatinosa, which is what small pain fibers do, opens the gate.

We are constantly bombarded by sensations of touch, position, pressure—sensations that run along large fibers. So the substantia gelatinosa is normally in a constant state of activity, and the pain gate is therefore normally closed to very minor pains—infinitesimal scratches or pricks. But when the pain is sharp enough to penetrate the normal activity of the substantia gelatinosa cells, it turns them off, allowing its noxious message to get through the gate to the T-cells and so on up into the brain.

Feeling pain, therefore, depends on the balance between the level of activity in our large fibers (which close the gate) and the level of pain carried by our small fibers (which open the gate).

But large fibers are fast, much faster than the small pain fibers. If you send a nonpain message, say, a vibrator touching your skin, it will get to the substantia gelatinosa faster than a pain message—a blow, a needle prick. And it will turn on the substantia gelatinosa neurons, closing the pain gate. This is something like tying up a telephone line by making calls when someone else wants to get through.

We do this to pain all the time. We rub or stroke a hurt, blow on a burn or bruise, scratch an itch. We stub a toe or crack a shin, and hop around, holding it. In doing this, we send fast nonpain messages in an attempt to close the gate and make the pain hurt less.

Before you take too much credit for so much knowledge of neurological mechanisms, consider the dog, the cat, or for that matter almost any animal. What does it do when it is injured? It licks the hurt area vigorously, sending nonpain messages to it spinal cord. All of us, animals and humans, have learned through experience that rubbing a hurt makes it feel better.

There is another influence on the gate, human, not animal, and that is the brain, which sends messages down into the spinal cord. There are fibers that extend from parts of the upper brain to the spinal cord, ending not very far from the substantia gelatinosa. These fibers, it is suggested, carry messages from the cerebral cortex—by definition, then, psychological messages—which raise or lower the sensitivity of the T-cells and of the neurons of the nearby spinal fibers.

This may be the mechanism by which the mind can actually turn off pain perception (as in the cases of the Anzio soldiers, the fire walkers, or the woman who believes in natural childbirth and objects to anesthesia). It's almost as if the cerebrum says to the substantia gelatinosa and the T-cells, "Pay no attention." Like the computer that flashes the code, "My inputs are clogged; no more information, please," the nervous system is capable of handling only a limited number of messages at any one time. If the system is "clogged" with nonpain messages, pain can't get through. And therefore does not hurt.

This system of balance between incoming pain and nonpain messages, plus messages coming down from the brain, is the pain gate hypothesis. It offers two new (and major) contributions to pain theory: the idea of *incoming* sensations inhibiting pain reception and the idea of a mechanism by which the *mind* inhibits pain reception.

It has practical implications. It offers explanations—and therefore suggests cures or at least treatments—for some of the long-standing pain puzzles we have already discussed. For example . . . .

In congenital analgesia the pain fibers entering the spinal cord are missing or defective at birth. The pain gate is permanently closed.

In prolonged pain the large fibers have been damaged by nerve disease and do not transmit their messages as fast, as frequently, or as often as normally. So the pain gate stays open longer, closes more slowly. Pain messages get through more easily, keep coming more frequently. Things hurt more and hurt for longer periods.

In hyperalgesia, extreme pain resulting from a normally nonpainful stimulus such as a light touch, a gentle vibration, the large fibers may have been entirely destroyed by nerve disease or other illness. The pain gate is always open; a scratch becomes torture.

Phantom limb pain requires a more complicated explanation. It is still an enormous mystery, but the pain gate hypothesis offers a possible explanation.

It seems that many, if not most, sufferers from phantom limb pain had severe pain in the same part of the missing limb *before* the amputation. It is rare to find such pain in soldiers who suddenly lose a healthy limb in combat or in previously healthy people who lose a limb as a result of accident. The phantom pain not only resembles but appears in the same place as the original pain.

Dr. Melzack describes the case of a patient who lost his hand during a period when he was suffering from a wooden splinter jammed under a fingernail of that hand. The man later complained of pain caused by a phantom splinter under a phantom nail in the phantom hand.

"It is possible," Dr. Melzack suggests, "that [such] prolonged pain may leave 'memory' traces . . ." in loops of cut nerve fiber. Normal inhibition of such memory traces is produced by the action of large fibers sending their close-the-gate sensations to the substantia gelatinosa.

The ends of the cut nerve fibers curl up in these loops and are intertwined with other tissues to form lumps of sensory axons in the stump of the amputated limb. These knots of nerve endings are still working, and since they are still connected to the rest of the nervous system, they send messages back to it, perhaps including "remembered" pain messages. Amputation destroys many large fibers and leaves others defective or inadequate, and this disturbance of the normal balance releases the "remembered" pain sensations from inhibition by opening the gate. "The release from inhibition," Dr. Melzack says, "could bring about activation of the [memory] traces to produce persistent, severe pain."

Probably, most influential has been the gate hypothesis' suggested explanation, for the first time, of how the mind controls and influences pain perception. It has been clear for some time that emotions, upbringing, attitudes, beliefs, and other psychological and social factors strongly color the way we react to pain. The gate hypothesis suggests the mechanisms by which they do this.

But the hypothesis and its supporters have not had everything their own way. There is considerable disagreement about the hypothesis and some opposition to it, even hostility among some researchers. Like all new ideas, it has provoked much debate and a great choosing of sides. This book cannot describe these differences in detail. But some of the questions raised by critics of the hypothesis can be briefly outlined.

For one thing, proof of the gate has yet to be established in the only way in which scientific data is ever established: through objective experimentation repeated successfully by others. It is true that large fibers are fast and conduct nonpain messages, and that pain fibers are slow and conduct pain messages. And it is true that fibers go from the brain—what messages they carry we do not know—down into the spinal cord. *But there is no evidence to prove that one kind of message opens or another closes the gate—or that there is any gate at all.*

Nor is there any evidence as to just how the neurons of the substantia gelatinosa function. Other nerve cells have been examined and recorded from—that is, their electric messages have been measured and evaluated—but no one has ever recorded from a substantia gelatinosa cell.

There have been some experiments in other laboratories that challenge Drs. Melzack and Wall's assumptions as to just how pain fibers influence neurons in the spinal cord. Some of these have been performed by scientists who themselves support the ideas of a gate control in the spinal cord. In summarizing these experiments, which suggest modifications in the gate hypothesis, Dr. Kenneth L. Casey of the University of Michigan concludes: "As additional experiments are performed under various conditions, it is likely that the complexity of intraspinal interactions will require further modifications of the gate hypothesis."

Dr. Melzack himself is quick to point out the cons as well as the pros. In a scientific paper published five years after the original hypothesis, he and Dr. Wall described new evidence that required modification of some of its details.

"The strength of the hypothesis," says Dr. Peter Sterling of the University of Pennsylvania, "is that it integrates a lot of facts. Its difficulty is that it is vague about precise neural mechanisms. . . . The hypothesis must be made more specific before it can be tested further. For one, it must state exactly how the various neurons in the thalamus control the flow of impulses. Not enough is known about the thalamus to make very good guesses."

It is in the field of clinical medicine, treating patients, that gate control has had its widest acceptance. This is because it seems to work, and as we have seen, doctors are practical people primarily concerned with what works and less concerned with explaining the mechanism by which it works.

Actually, people have relieved one pain by causing another for centuries. The application of mustard plasters, ice packs, hot-water bottles, and other forms of what used to be called counterirritation goes back many years in folk medicine. It is still in use today.

This concept of relieving pain by raising the level of non-pain sensation—sending messages to the substantia gelatinosa that will close the pain gate—had also been observed by earlier pain researchers. About ten years before Drs. Melzack and Wall published their paper, Dr. Sumner Trent, then of New York's Psychiatric Hospital, described a merchant seaman who had suffered a head injury. As a result of brain damage, he experienced unexplained, almost continuous, pain over his entire right arm and hand. He also felt as if his arm were burning, and he suffered unbearable pain (hyperalgesia) when the doctor pricked his skin lightly with a needle.

"The pain was completely eliminated," Dr. Trent reported, "by pressure on the tips of the four fingers of his right hand. During the examination the patient exerted this pressure by grasping his left arm or knee, or by clenching his right fist. The hyperalgesia to pinprick completely and immediately disappeared when pressure was put on the fingergips of the right hand."

In the summer of 1972, seventeen years later, Dr. Trent

wrote in a letter to *Science* magazine that in his opinion the case was later explained by the gate control hypothesis.

Since the gate idea was born it has in turn given birth to new ideas about curing pain. One of these is the concept of electrical stimulation, in which an electric current is sent along the large fibers to close the pain gate. This has been done successfully in many cases of severe intractable pain that could not be cured by surgery or by pain-killing drugs.

Another may be the Chinese practice of acupuncture. It may be that the acupuncturist's needles work by sending strong pressure and vibration messages to close the gate. But here the hypothesis is on shakier ground, and it is not entirely clear that this is what happens during acupuncture. Yet gate control has encouraged the clinical use of, and further research in, acupuncture for analgesia.

Some pain treatments work through the power of the mind to send analgesic messages down to the gate. Hypnosis is not new, but there is a strange new approach called biofeedback.

All of these treatment methods—electrostimulation, acupuncture, hypnosis, biofeedback—will be described later in this book. First let us mention an important research direction that the gate control hypothesis has opened up: the search for better pain-relieving drugs.

"Better" in that sentence means not only more effective but also less addictive, if not nonaddictive. At the present time the very best analgesic drug known to man is morphine or its legal derivatives. Its illegal derivative, heroin, is pretty good, too. The problem with these is well known. Other analgesic drugs, sedatives, and tranquilizers also have addictive side effects.

The gate control hypothesis suggests possible new ways in which drugs might operate. Present pain-killers work by turning off parts of the brain or parts of the spinal cord. Researchers may find new drugs that work by decreasing the effect of small fibers or increasing the effect of large fibers on

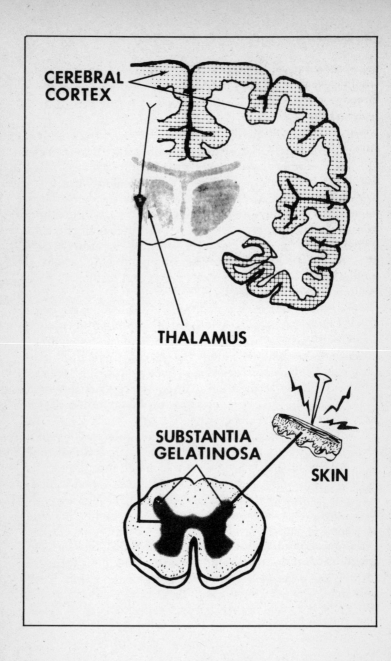

CEREBRAL CORTEX

THALAMUS

SUBSTANTIA GELATINOSA

SKIN

the substantia gelatinosa. Either or both of these actions would close the pain gate. Or they may find drugs that work directly on the substantia gelatinosa. Its cells are known to resist all the stains (necessary for microscope viewing) that work with other neurons. This suggests that the chemistry of substantia gelatinosa neurons may be very different from that of other neurons. If this is in fact the case, a drug may be developed that works only on the substantia gelatinosa. Such a drug might possibly have none of the unpleasant, dangerous, or addictive system-wide effects of other analgesic drugs.

So far we have been talking of pain as a unity. But all pains do not hurt the same, are not caused by identical mechanisms, are not soothed by similar treatments. A headache is not a toothache. Neither is it a sprained ankle. The pain of childbirth, with which life outside the womb begins, is not a heart attack, which ends many lives. Menstrual cramps are not charley horses.

Let us now see where it hurts—and why.

Figure 6. A simplified sketch of pain pathways, taking into consideration the gate hypothesis. The impulse produced by an unpleasant stimulus travels along sensory fibers to the gate in the substantia gelatinosa in the spinal cord, across the cord to the white matter on the other side, and up the cord to the thalamus. Complex interactions between the thalamus and the cerebral cortex result, in some as yet unknown way, in the *perception* of the impulse as pain, and in the *reactions* to that pain. The cortex can also send impulses to the thalamus and down the spinal cord to "close the gate," blocking reception of pain messages.

Chapter 9

The Most Common Pain: Headache

Something like 90 percent of all pain is headache pain, making it humanity's most common medical complaint. And no doubt one of its most tormenting. "When the head aches," wrote Cervantes in *Don Quixote*, "all the members partake of the pains." Most headaches are caused by events going on in the muscles or blood vessels *outside* the skull, and not by diseases or injuries *inside* the brain or the brain's cavity.

The trick is to reassure oneself that the vast majority of all headaches are outside jobs, even if they hurt as if a bull is loose inside the china shop of your mind. Not many headaches are caused by brain tumors or other inside horrors.

It's not always reassuring to remember this, however. If pain in general is subjective—something only *you* can feel —headache pain is more so. Doctors can't X-ray it, can't take its temperature, can't diagnose it by blood test or microscope, and a tumor headache doesn't necessarily feel different from the ordinary kind. You tell the doctor how your head feels, and he tells you—if he's clever and lucky, and you're lucky—what it's caused by, usually something you can live with. Few headaches last very long; few need a doctor's care; most are easily relieved with aspirin.

The vast majority are caused either by muscle tension or by blood vessel expansion or contraction outside the skull. These are best described as "tension" headaches. They are far and away the most common, as well as the most harmless, even if they do hurt pretty badly. The worse thing that can be said about them is that they hurt and are responsible for the most stupid, boring, and misleading of television commercials.

The important word is "tension," because this is what causes them and this is what distinguishes them from migraine headaches or more serious headache problems. The tension is emotional or "nervous," take your choice, and is caused by fatigue, frustration, worry, overwork, anger, etc., in any combination or alone.

Most tension headaches are muscle-contraction headaches, and they hurt because the muscles of the face, forehead, scalp, and neck—all or some of them—are in a prolonged or constant state of contraction. Try grinning for more than thirty seconds, and you'll get a small idea of what happens when the muscles around your skull stay tight for very long.

No one knows exactly how tension causes these head muscles to tighten up. It may be that the overstimulation of nerve fibers by anxiety or some other psychological state results in an overload of nerve impulses, and that these impulses then "spill over" to trigger an exaggerated muscle response.

A common mechanism of tension headache is contraction of the muscle that lies across the forehead. This is the muscle we contract to wrinkle the brow or move the eyebrows up or down. In many tension states this muscle contracts imperceptibly, little by little, until it has tightened up to the point of headache.

The great German playwright and poet Bertolt Brecht wrote a brief and amusing poem about angry, or "bad" or "evil," thoughts as a cause of this kind of pain.

The Mask of Evil

On my wall hangs a Japanese carving,
The mask of an evil demon, decorated with gold lacquer.

Sympathetically I observe
The swollen veins of the forehead, indicating
What a strain it is to be evil.

The pain of muscle headaches is steady, does not throb or pulse, and is usually (though not always) located on both sides or in the center of the head. It can come and go, move around, leave and return. Or it can stay for weeks or even months. It can be a dull ache at the back of the head or it can feel like a band around the top of the head, like cramps, or like a vise tightened at the temples.

The best treatment is aspirin. Massage, rest, warmth, and hot baths also help. So does the passage of time; sometimes one can just lie down and wait—if one can wait long enough—for it to go away. In very severe cases, when headaches of this type are long-lasting or constantly recurring, doctors will prescribe mood-changing drugs—tranquilizers, sedatives, or antidepressants. Treat these drugs with caution and suspicion. They should be taken only as a last resort; unlike aspirin, they are addictive and can probably do more harm to your health than the headache. While the headache may make you *want* to die, it can't do you any real harm.

Does liquor help? Insofar as alcohol is probably the best and the most pleasant of the mood-changing drugs (some prefer marijuana) and may even be better for you than its chemical relatives, the sedatives and tranquilizers, it may in mild cases relax the tension enough to relieve the headache. Two cautions, though: one, alcohol is addictive, and too much steady use can lead to you know what; and two, the headache of a hangover is no improvement over that of tension. For really bad, chronic tension headaches, alcohol is a no-no.

Not all tension headaches are caused by muscle reactions. The blood vessels also respond with great sensitivity to nervous system impulses, and so the other mechanical cause of headache pain is narrowing or expanding of the blood vessels outside the skull. This sudden pressure on the wall of the arteries and capillaries *hurts*. (Vascular pressure or twisting is a common cause of pain from inside the body. The pain of various forms of heart attack, for example, comes from sudden blockage of, or pressure on, blood vessels. Tie a cord around your arm tight enough to stop the circulation and you will feel vascular pain.)

The mechanism by which tension causes these changes in the blood vessels of the scalp, forehead, and temples is not much better understood than that of muscle contraction. It may be that the overflow of nerve impulses, already mentioned as the possible cause of muscles' tightening, also affects nearby blood vessels.

What is more likely is that a sudden change in the body's chemistry is responsible. Stress of any kind causes drastic change in the release of hormones, the body's chemical messengers. Powerful emotions in the cerebral cortex and thalamus (fear, hatred, anger, sexual excitement, anxiety) influence the hypothalamus, a tiny section of the brain which regulates the body's normal chemical balance and the functioning of the sympathetic nervous system. The hypothalamus, for example, is responsible for our sweating when we are excited. It also directs the adrenal glands to release its hormones, which affect the caliber of blood vessels. This in turn may produce sufficient vascular constriction to cause headache.

While some tension headaches are caused by these blood vessel changes, most vascular headaches fall into the special category of migraine. In migraine the pain is produced by the same painful tightening of arteries and capillaries as in tension headaches, but migraine is a different type of headache, with rather unusual qualities.

Migraine is common, ancient, and mysterious. Speaking conservatively, from 5 to 10 percent of Americans—that adds up to 10 to 20 million people—suffer from one or another form of migraine. Not that it's an "American" affliction; millions of sufferers are found all over the world, and have existed in all periods of history.

Migraine has been around since man and woman began their history, and probably before that. Hippocrates, the ancient Greek father of medicine, who lived more than twenty-four hundred years ago, wrote about it. Julius Caesar had it. So did Saint Paul and countless other historic figures.

A bit more than a century after the time of Jesus Christ, a Greek physician named Aretaeus described it in these remarkably accurate terms:

> The pain is sometimes on the right, and sometimes on the left side, of the forehead. . . . [It is] an illness by no means mild. . . . It occasions unseemly and dreadful symptoms . . . nausea, vomiting . . . collapse . . . and life becomes a burden. For they flee the light; the darkness soothes their disease . . . the patients are weary of life and wish to die.

A migraine is like no other headache. Some distinctive features of these vascular attacks are caused by sudden dilatation of one or another of the arteries supplying the head and brain. In addition to the swelling of these blood vessels, pain is also caused by the associated accumulation and pressure of fluid in the tissues immediately surrounding them.

The special features of migraine include first of all its periodic nature; migraine attacks occur at fairly regular intervals, as close as once a month, as far apart as once or twice a year. These attacks are also paroxysmal; they are sudden and violent.

You don't keep on doing what you're doing when you have a migraine attack; you are overcome with a sudden need to find some dark, quiet place, crawl into it like the sick animal you are, and stay there until the migraine goes away. In fact this is what most sufferers do, and it often works.

Migraines last in most cases from several hours to one or two days. The pain is throbbing, and rhythmic, and as these pains progress, they merge into one constant, steady pain. There is often nausea, vomiting, dizziness, irritability, and unpleasant reactions to bright lights. Migraine almost always occurs on one or the other side of the head (the term comes from the word for "half-skull" in Greek), usually around the temples. It is much more common among women than among men, and since it runs in families, it may be hereditary. It's really a form of disease, rather than a headache. Often starting before the teen-age years, it stays for life. But if it hasn't begun before age forty-five, it probably never will.

Certain events occur prior to a migraine attack. Experienced sufferers recognize these events as a warning and take whatever medication they have, find that dark room to lie down in, or try to follow the new techniques of biofeedback. Biofeedback has been found to be very helpful in treating headaches, and more will be said about it in Chapter 18. These early warnings, which an alert and trained patient can recognize, are caused by changes in the circulation. The arteries in the head expand and contract with some instability, and the sufferer will alternately experience flushing and paleness, as well as occasional dizziness. His or her hands and feet may appear cold and clammy, because blood is beginning to move from these extremities to the vessels in the head.

There appears to be some kind of inverse cardiovascular relationship between the hands and feet and the head, so that when one is full of blood and warm, the other is emptied of blood and cold. To the old saying "Cold hands, warm heart," one may add a new version for migraine people: "Cold hands, warm head, and now is the time to lie down in that dark, quiet place!"

Hand temperature just before a migraine attack has been found to drop from normal of about 90° F. to as low as 70° F. Thermographs (heat pictures) of the brain during a migraine attack have shown a drop in skin temperature as blood rushes inward to swell the arteries close to the skull and brain.

The most spectacular aspect of migraine, occurring in about 15 percent of all attacks, is the aura. An aura is a sensory message that appears regularly just before the migraine, as a kind of premonitory warning. It can be a feeling, a smell, or most often a visual experience. In some migraines the sufferer sees lights or geometric structures or perhaps thinks he or she is looking at the world through the wrong end of a microscope. One migraine sufferer "smelled" ammonia before her attacks. Another "felt" a sudden rush of cold air up into her head.

Most mild migraines can be handled with a day or so of rest and aspirin. Really crippling migraine pain is treated with a drug that constricts the blood vessels and sends the blood back down from the skull. This medicine is a derivative of the chemical ergot, and can be taken by mouth, suppository, or injection. It is often combined with caffeine, the drug found in coffee. This medicine seems to help, but ergot is dangerous for patients who have high blood pressure, heart disease, kidney disease, or liver disease, or are pregnant.

Some women are very much helped by doses of the female sex hormone progesterone. A number of women find that their migraines appear to coincide with menstrual periods, and might be called menstrual migraine. This may be because just prior to the beginning of menstruation, there is a very rapid rise in levels of the other female hormone, estrogen, and then a sudden drop. This rapid fluctuation in estrogen is believed to cause rapid changes in blood vessel dilatation and contraction. In fact some women who suffer ordinary headaches when they take oral contraceptives may be suffering from a similar effect, since the pills contain synthetic versions of estrogen.

Many women see their migraines disappear during pregnancy, when there is an enormous increase in progesterone in the blood. Progesterone may counteract estrogen and relieve migraine pain.

Women sometimes find that their migraines disappear after a number of years and then come back during or just after the menopause. The menopause is caused first by a sudden and permanent drop in progesterone, and followed by a similar and more significant decline in estrogen. Even women without migraine may suffer flashes, dizziness, and headaches as a result of these changes in the body's blood chemistry at middle age.

What triggers migraines? Most researchers agree that migraine people are often a special type: anxious, hardworking, ambitious, perfectionist, and rigid. When migraine people are faced with conflict or frustration, they tend to become tense, tired, and a bit angry. All these psychological states, developing in the cerebral cortex, have a profound effect on the hypothalamus, the switchboard that does for outgoing brain messages what the thalamus does for incoming. The theory is that the hypothalamus, which regulates the mechanisms of body chemistry, translates these cerebral tension messages into blood vessel messages of contraction and dilatation.

Many migraine sufferers will say that yes, their attacks do come at fairly regular periods, but that there is always something exhausting or upsetting to trigger the event—a long automobile drive or a crisis in the office or a frustrating family quarrel.

With the increasing specialization in health care, we now have not only headache clinics (Montefiore Hospital, New York) and pain clinics (University of Washington Hospital, Seattle) but also the world's first migraine clinic. This is the Princess Margaret Migraine Clinic of London, sponsored by Britain's Migraine Trust.

Most migraine sufferers don't see a doctor until after the attack is well under way or has gone. But at the Princess Margaret Clinic (she suffers from migraine), free (for Britons) emergency treatment is given to patients during their migraine attacks.

When a patient feels a migraine attack coming on, he or she can walk into Princess Margaret and find a physician, a nursing staff, and a comfortable bed in a quiet, darkened room. The physician offers the patient medication, including a pain-killer and an antivomiting drug, and leaves the patient alone to lie down and relax. The nurse calls the patient's employer or home to report what has happened, or does whatever else is practical. Eight out of every ten patients who walk in during business hours return to work or home that same day or early the next morning. If the patient is too sick to get home alone, the clinic pays for a cab.

Because the clinic treats patients *during* the attack, its staff is able to carry out important research about how migraine affects sufferers and how it is relieved by treatment. Out of this research may come a new approach to treatment that is safe for patients with heart trouble or high blood pressure.

Neither tension nor migraine headaches are threats to life; one sees a doctor for relief rather than for cure. How can one tell whether one had, in fact, one of these two common headaches or some more threatening kind—a headache caused by a disease process? What is the rule of thumb distinguishing danger-signal headaches from tension and migraine headaches? Here are the warning signs of headaches that mean more than tension or migraine:

1. Headache accompanied by fever, convulsions, pain in the eye or ear, or disorientation and unconsciousness.

2. Headache coming after a blow.

3. Sudden, unexplainable headache, especially if it is very severe.

Don't panic. A doctor can't always tell, but he can, if he's any good at all, tell more easily than you can. And don't let your doctor panic you. Brain tumors are rare. Dr. J. Lawrence Pool, a famous Columbia University neurosurgeon, now retired, tells the story, in his excellent book *Your Brain and Nerves*, of a young woman patient sent to him by a psychiatrist.

Before seeing the psychiatrist, this young woman was tormented by a severe headache at the top and back of her head for three months. Examinations and X rays showed nothing. She began to take pain-killing drugs and in time became addicted to them. Her suffering led her to attempt suicide, and she was finally referred to the psychiatrist. When he could find nothing wrong, he sent her to Dr. Pool's clinic for brain surgery!

But Dr. Pool, who is apparently wise as well as kind, guessed that even though he could find no physical cause, her pain probably had some physical origin other than a brain tumor. He suspected a sinus problem and sent her to the Columbia University Medical Center's nose and throat specialist. The specialist discovered, and removed, a quantity of pus that had been blocking one of her sinuses. Her headache vanished that same day.

Not all headaches end so happily. But the ones that arise because of such serious problems as brain tumors or blood clots in the brain's blood vessels are rare. They sometimes manifest themselves as headaches at the center of the forehead; more often they cause no pain at all. As we know, brain tissue is not sensitive to pain.

A rare but painful form of head pain is caused by disease of one of the nerve fibers serving the head—the trigeminal or fifth cranial nerve, a three-branched fiber that conveys sensation from the chin, the cheek, and the forehead. One, two, or three of the branches may be affected by disease, which has no known cause. The stabbing, terrible pains of trigeminal neuralgia (it is also called *tic douloureux,* which in French means "painful spasm") start at the throat and spread up to the ear. The pain is so bad it has driven sufferers—usually people over fifty, more often women than men—to drug addiction, alcoholism, and suicide.

Chapter 10

The Most Sensitive Organ: The Mouth

The mouth must be one of the most vulnerable organs. No threat to the body evokes more fright and anxiety than a threat to the mouth, especially to the teeth. Young and old appear to be more frightened of the dentist's drill than of the surgeon's knife.

Evidence of the overwhelming psychological nature of dental pain is the fact that until a few years ago approximately one-fifth of all administrations of general anesthesia in the United States were ordered not by surgeons but by dentists. People who can face abdominal incisions with no more protection than the needle of regional or local anesthesia will often insist that they be "knocked out" before the dentist starts his drill. Fear of the dentist is powerful enough to keep millions of patients who need dental care from getting it. (There are, of course, other reasons in addition to fear that keep people from the dentist.)

Perhaps it is because the mouth is part of the head, the place where the real self is thought to exist, the site of the brain, face, and personality. My stomach is only my faceless gut, but what I see in the mirror is the *real* me. Perhaps it is because from birth the mouth is our earliest and most important source of pleasure and satisfaction.

"Many adults," a psychiatrist comments,

continue to find their pleasure mainly in its use, as in eating, drinking, smoking, or sexual enjoyment. Pain in this area seems to be especially resented. Often, too, there are specific problems about having the mouth immobilized, because of its use in eating and breathing, and . . . as a primitive weapon of defense—used in biting, yelling, talking back.

Fear of dental pain—whether the pain is caused by tooth or mouth disease or by its treatment—may be based largely on psychological states rather than physical causes because there seems to be less of a neurological structure to carry pain messages from teeth than from other parts of the body. Teeth are not well supplied with the neurons that receive pain signals, although there are nerve fibers that carry such signals to the spinal cord and brain. In fact, dental researchers are still not sure how and why we feel pain when our teeth are drilled or when exposed dentin is touched by heat or cold, by sweet or sour fluids, or by food or air.

The outside of the tooth, the part that we see, is composed of enamel. This is hard, dead, protective "armor" consisting almost entirely of the mineral calcium. It has no neurons, no nerve fibers, no blood vessels.

The bulk of the tooth protected by this outer covering is made of dentin, a partly calcium tissue which has no blood vessels, and probably no nerve fibers, although there is controversy over this. Some researchers say dentin is not penetrated by any nerve fibers; others say that it may have a few, projecting into tiny fjordlike channels. The great mystery is how dentin transmits pain.

For it is through the dentin that pain travels when you have a cavity—a wearing away, or cracking of, or opening in the enamel. Exposure of the dentin to almost any stimulus is perceived as pain.

Inside the dentin is where your tooth "lives." Here in the pulp, a soft tissue, as its name indicates, is a supply of blood vessels and nerve fibers. This pulp is understandably sensitive to pain, although it is not usually involved in the more common types of dental problems. When it is, as in abscesses or other disease processes, it sends pain messages in the usual manner, unless the sensory neurons have been destroyed. The pulp forms a core, extending down into the root of the tooth, where its tiny blood vessels and nerve fibers join the artery and nerve fiber that runs along the jaw.

That nerve fiber, a branch of the trigeminal nerve, rings the jawbone until it enters other branches in the gradually thickening fiber in the neck. The trigeminal nerve is one of the cranial nerves.

Exactly how stimuli produce pain messages through enamel and dentin is not known. Researchers have advanced many theories, none of which is yet entirely accepted.

But dentists know very well the origin of specific dental pains, even if their mechanisms are unclear. And dentists know how to evaluate and treat the pains' underlying disease conditions. Such conditions should be treated, not only because they can, if left to themselves, cause even greater pain, but also because they can lead to serious and irreversible destruction of teeth, gums, or bone tissue.

Most tooth pain serves the useful function of warning us that a tooth has been attacked and is threatened with decay, its most common enemy. Decay is believed to come from outside, caused by the action of bacteria in the mouth. These bacteria, which are there all the time, have the ability to convert sugar into an acid that can eat away at enamel and dentin. This is why sugar is poison to teeth. There are other theories as to the origin of tooth decay.

By the time such decay has eaten a cavity into dentin, the pain can be pretty bad, because a sensitive area has been exposed to chemical, pressure, or temperature changes. If decay goes deeper, the result may be an abscess inside the tooth. In addition to the pain produced by exposure of the dentin, an abscess, which is completely enclosed in the tooth, produces pus or gas. The pressure of either of these against the nerve fibers can produce severe pain.

Tooth pain must be heeded because of the progressive destruction that decay can cause. It is wise to have a dental checkup periodically, in order to have cavities filled and decay arrested *before* it has gone so far as to cause pain.

The gums provide other pathways for infection that can produce toothache. If bacteria cause infections down between the gum or bone and the root of the tooth, such pressure-producing abscesses can also cause pain. So can inflammation of a gum flap over an erupting or badly positioned (impacted) wisdom tooth.

Less common but no less painful is a cracked tooth. Sometimes, although the crack may be almost invisible, the pain can be excruciating. A cracked tooth hurts most during chewing or biting. The pain is caused by pressure and vibration traveling down the crack to the nerve fiber in the pulp.

Some pain is caused by a poorly fitting metal restoration. Metal is an excellent conductor of heat and cold (as well as of electric current), and if the gold inlay or silver amalgam, or the backing or lining the dentist puts under it, has deteriorated or was improperly set, the metal can relay painful sensations through the dentin to the nerve fiber in the pulp. One can experience the same pain in healthy teeth if one tries to bite into a piece of ice.

And then, of course, there is the pain that is caused by the dentist.

There is now much less dental pain than there used to be. Much pain was caused in the past by the heat and vibration of the drill on enamel. But now with newer high-speed drills which vibrate very much less, this pain has been reduced and even sometimes eliminated. Newer and better equipment promises to reduce this pain even further.

There are also anesthetic drugs which can be injected to block the unavoidable pain caused by the dentist's work. These are commonly used during extractions, during drilling into dentin or close to the pulp, and during work on the root canals of the teeth or other kinds of dental surgery. The drug—most often either procaine or lidocaine—is injected into the jaw as close as possible to the nerve.

This anesthetic interferes—for a certain period of time, depending upon which drug is used and how much is injected—with the ability of the neurons to transmit messages. No messages can then be transmitted from the nerve to the brain. The result is a feeling of numbness in the general area of the tooth, gum, cheek, and mouth during which the dentist can do his work without the patient feeling any sensation. By the time the drug wears off, the pain is usually bearable. If not, aspirin or some other mild analgesic drug can block the remaining pain sensation.

Nitrous oxide, the gas often used for general anesthesia in dentistry, or Pentothal, an injectable anesthetic, can be given in limited quantities so as to put the patient into a light sleep during which pain is reduced. Full dosages bring unconsciousness. Little dental work requires general anesthesia, despite the many requests for it, and in recent years dentists have increasingly turned to light sedation instead.

And dentists, perhaps mindful of those many requests and the unreasoning fear they express, have been conscious of, and open to, new ways of blocking pain. Dentists are probably more experimental-minded about pain than physicians, who do not face the problem as often. Among these newer ways are analgesic sprays which briefly "deaden" pain receptor neurons in the skin surface so that the anesthetc needle doesn't hurt. More sensational have been the occasional use of hypnosis, acupuncture, and audio analgesia to block pain.

Hypnosis and acupuncture are discussed in later chapters. But a word about audio analgesia, the use of sound as a pain-killer, may be in order.

In 1959 dental researchers published a report in the *Journal of the American Dental Association* describing the use of sound to kill the pain of drilling and pulling teeth. It was quickly labeled audio analgesia.

To a profession constantly plagued with the problem of pain and the guilt of contributing to that pain, and to those who make a profit selling gadgets to dentists, the idea of playing sound recordings and stereophonic music as a pain-killer seemed to be a sensational leap forward. Audio analgesia was greeted with excitement and enthusiasm. It certainly appeared superior to sticking drug-filled needles into people or "putting them to sleep." Companies jumped into the business of making and selling high-fidelity and stereo equipment specially designed for the dental office. These were equipped with headsets and tone and volume controls for the patient.

Many dentists bought them. Some had dramatic successes. A few patients said that when the sets were tuned in, they felt no pain during either drilling or extraction.

But others said it had no effect on their pain. And those for whom audio analgesia worked at one time found that it did not always work at other times.

Further studies showed that in the hands of a highly per-suasive dentist with a compelling, take-charge personality, audio analgesia could work. Dentist who had doubts and were not high-pressure salesmen, found they could not use it very successfully. Matter-of-fact dentists who merely put the headset on the patient and reached for the drill found it did not work for them, either.

The patient's personality was a factor. Some people are more easily manipulated than others. Such patients, in the hands of a domineering dentist, could be "talked into" using the audio analgesia successfully. Success with this method, therefore, had more to do with the personality of dentist and patient than with the method itself. This is also the chief shortcoming with hypnosis.

Dr. Ronald Melzack and his associates studied audio analgesia in laboratory experiments with volunteers, not with real patients, and found that it probably wasn't "analgesia" at all but a form of attention distraction. The music diverted the patient's attention away from the pain. It kept the brain "busy" listening and keeping time, while the pain message sneaked (so to speak) into the brain. The cerebral cortex wasn't "looking," it was "listening" to music.

Audio analgesia never had a chance. It was too unreliable, too expensive, and too complicated. Needles remained the method of deadening most dental pain, and the expensive hi-fi sets and stereo headsets went, as Dr. Melzack puts it, "to the attic of dental history."

"The story of 'audio analgesia,'" he concluded, "contains an important moral: there is no easy, magical relief for pain."

Pain is both useful in and a special problem of dental diagnosis. It is *useful* because, by calling attention to the location and nature of the problem, it helps the dentist determine the source—which tooth, and whether it is caused by cavity, abscess of tooth or gums, loose or damaged filling, or impacted wisdom tooth. It is a *problem* because of pain referral in, to, and from the mouth—a very common occurrence.

In Chapter 4 the printer whose toothache was referred to his chest is described. So also is the tragic case of the man whose heart pain masqueraded as toothache.

Sometimes pain may be referred to a tooth from an ear or even from what may turn out to be a brain tumor. A dentist has to be an astute observer and an acute listener to make sure that some nondental pain is not presenting itself in the guise of a toothache.

In most dental pain referrals, the dentist is confronted with pain in one tooth when, in fact, the abscess or the pulp decay is in a different tooth. Such referred pain rarely crosses the midline of the body; if the disease is in a tooth on the left side of the mouth, the pain will be referred to another tooth on that side and will almost never cross to the opposite side. But it can be referred from an infection in a bottom tooth to a tooth in the top jaw.

In addition to taking a careful history of the pain—where it started, when it started, if it moved, under what condition it seemed to move, whether it was throbbing or steady—the dentist has certain tools to help him in his detective work. He can take X rays, and these can show him where the actual problem is. He can also tap each tooth lightly and note what effect, if any, this has on the pain.

Electrical pulp testing is often used to locate the tooth with a pulp problem. The dentist sends a tiny electric current through each tooth. By measuring the voltage required to bring forth a response from the patient, he can tell if the pulp is healthy or not. A healthy pulp will respond to current; a diseased or dead one will not.

But this technique is not always accurate, because it can be affected by all sorts of variables, such as the patient's age, emotional outlook, or how thick or worn his tooth enamel is. Even when these variables are accounted for, dead pulp will sometimes seem to respond, and healthy pulp will not.

Some dentists find heat tests more accurate than electrical. Something that produces heat, or a heated instrument, is touched to each tooth. If the tooth is healthy, the patient will feel pain, but the pain will disappear a few seconds after the heat is removed. If the pain is extreme, the dentist will suspect pulp disease in that particular tooth. On the other hand, cold will hurt healthy teeth, but not those that are diseased.

Or the dentist can press his finger on the bottom of each tooth, where it enters the gum, and ask the patient to open and close. If the patient winces at one tooth, that tooth has a problem.

Local anesthetic can also be a useful diagnostic tool. After injecting a very small amount of the drug near a suspected tooth, the dentist can then see if the pain goes away. If it does, the pain came from that particular tooth.

Toothache is one of those few pains that does its duty as a warning signal. This is so rarely the case with other major pains that perhaps we should be grateful and heed its warning. It's an excellent reason to go to the dentist, a poor one for staying away.

But even in dentistry *absence* of pain is not foolproof evidence that nothing is wrong. Tooth and gum disease can be very advanced, too far advanced for treatment, without any pain warning signal.

Chapter 11

The Pain of Being Human: Backache

We are the only animal that walks erect, and we pay a price in pain for this distinction. Our grandparents called it backache or lumbago. Nowadays doctors call it low back pain.

Back pain has much in common with headache. Like headache, it is often caused by muscle spasms resulting from fatigue and/or tension. Like headache, it can be a vague and nagging pain that defies diagnosis and resists treatment. And like headache, it too can be caused by infection or disease not directly related to the location of the pain. No one has actually counted, but it is believed that a great many patients have been mistakenly shunted off to psychiatrists or surgeons by impatient doctors frustrated by their own inability to cure headache or backache.

The trouble with the human back is the load it has to bear plus the jobs it has to do. It has to be strong enough to carry most of our weight, and yet so flexible that it can bend forward and down almost in a perfect U, sideways approaching an angle of forty-five degrees, and backwards in a small but significant arc. (Gymnasts and acrobats can get even greater performance from their spines.) In addition, the backbone protects with its bony armor the vital spinal cord, as well as the roots of all the nerve fibers coming into that cord.

Achieving this strength and flexibility is a spine constructed of twenty-four individual segments of bone, called vertebrae, hinged to each other by interlocking bony projections. They are further held together by ligaments and other muscular and connecting tissues. Running through a hole in each vertebra is the vital spinal cord.

Each vertebra is separated from the one above and below it by a kind of shock absorber, a disk of cartilage, a tough material, looking and feeling something like a thick oyster. If the disk were not there, every time we moved our back one bony vertebra would grind against another. Instead, the friction is taken up by this soft, flexible cushion. As we grow older, this cushion loses its moisture, thickness, and flexibility. But it may also lose these early in life, even in the teens. Or the disk can push or "slip" out of place as a result of some sudden action, during a tennis set, for example. If, when this happens, the disk presses against a nerve root, we feel pain.

These things usually happen in the disks that bear the most strain and weight and take the greatest amount of mechanical punishment. The disks most vulnerable are those between the five lowest vertebrae in the small of the back. Hence "low back" pain. Disk difficulties can also occur in the seven vertebrae of the neck, as in the "whiplash" injury that follows many automobile accidents when the head snaps back and forth suddenly.

Another common source of back pain is tension of the muscles and ligaments connecting the vertebrae to each other and to other bones of the skeleton. Just as anxiety and fatigue cause the muscles of the scalp and forehead and neck to tighten, so also do they cause the muscles of the back to tighten. The way we sit, stand, or drive a car can contribute to this tightening. So can the unconsciously rigid way we hold ourselves when we are nervous or tense.

Years ago, when most people spent their lives in physical work, back muscles were exercised more often and remained supple and loose longer. But almost all of us today do work that requires us to sit or stand in more or less one position. We do much less physical work, and we do less physical activity in our play. The automobile is probably the greatest contributor to low back pain because we rarely walk much anymore, and walking is one of the best forms of exercise for the more than one hundred muscles involved in keeping the backbone straight and in controlling its movements.

Most back pain is tension- or disk-caused. But as with headache, one often worries at first that it might be caused by something more serious. A persistent backache can be produced by almost any disease within the body, from a kidney stone stuck in the ureter to a growth in a woman's womb. Even a lung cancer can press against the tissues of the back and be felt as back pain.

But fortunately, most back pain is just that, and can be treated, if it is caused by muscle tension or spasm, by various kinds of relaxants. These can be a warm bath or a warm massage or just putting warm, wet towels on the sore part. Aspirin works fine too. Some rest is good, but not too much, and it should be followed by gentle stretching exercises.

Disk pain can be pretty bad. An out-of-place disk that presses on the sciatic nerve—the longest nerve in the body, running from the "tail" of the spine down into the foot—is sheer torture.

In the past disk pain was treated by rest and traction—pulling the top and bottom parts of the body apart by the use of weights and pulleys, so that the vertebrae separate slightly, and pressure on the disk is reduced. Some form of pain-killing drug was also usually given.

But this didn't always work, and so surgery to remove the part of the disk pressing against the nerve root was—and still is—often done as a last resort. Even this doesn't always work, either. In really bad cases surgeons will fuse the two vertebrae together with pegs of bone, so that they do not move. This is a risky operation with a number of serious hazards, and the welding doesn't always work.

Now a newly discovered chemical is being tried instead of surgery. The chemical, an enzyme similar to meat tenderizer, is injected directly into the protruding disk through long needles. It softens, shrinks, and even dissolves the swollen portion of the disk that is pressing on the nerve root.

Back pain is with us, probably to stay. Our spine is designed for four-footed animals, and since we humans persist in standing and walking erect, this bony, flexible structure will no doubt persist in suffering special stress and strain.

Chapter 12

Women and Pain

Women suffer an extra pain burden and not because they have "lower pain thresholds"; they don't.

All human societies put women down in many ways, and one is by labeling them weak, complaining, self-pitying creatures. A woman's pain counts for less than a man's. Her suffering is taken less seriously.

A complaining old man, for example, is usually described as "an old woman." A boy or a man who stands up to pain with little or no complaint is "manly." If he does not, if he cries and whimpers, he is a "sissy" or a "faggot."

The result of this prejudice is that since women and girls are *expected* to cry and complain, less attention is paid to them. Their complaints are often dismissed as "not real," "all in the head," "nervousness."

Doctors, almost all of whom are men, express the same prejudice when they do not take seriously such specifically female complaints as menstrual pains. Sometimes, when they label these pains "emotional" or "psychosomatic," they seem to be telling a woman that her cramps don't really exist.

But *all* pain exists *if it is felt*. Dr. Audrey McMaster of the Oklahoma University School of Medicine answered those who dismiss female pain when she read this limerick at the annual meeting of the American College of Obstetricians and Gynecologists in 1974:

There was a young lady from Deal,
Who said, "Although pain isn't real,
    When I sit on a pin
    And it punctures my skin
I dislike what I fancy I feel."

Women conditioned to see themselves in a weak, self-pitying light often try to please by agreeing that their pains are not important. They think it is their duty to be uncomplaining, especially about "female" problems. "Female" pains don't count; it is considered "normal" to have them; women should "expect" to put up with menstrual cramps.

Some women have begun to question and to challenge this downgrading of their pains. They do not want to suffer in silence, and they refuse to be put off by a doctor's offhand dismissal. They are not accepting the notion that their pain "isn't really there," that it's a psychiatric or emotional problem. Partly as a result of the women's liberation movement, female patients are today pressing doctors to deal with their pain problems with the same respect accorded *other* pain problems. Pelvic pain, they say, hurts just as much and is just as important medically as chest pain or back pain.

Emotions and personality and one's rearing as a female do, of course, have an important influence on how one perceives and responds to pain. While one woman can have a perfectly painless childbirth without any anesthetic, another may suffer so much pain she needs to be put asleep by general anesthesia. Such emotional states as her attitude toward the unborn baby, toward motherhood, and toward her husband can affect the degree of pain she may feel. Certainly, menstrual pain may also be affected by a woman's attitudes toward menstruation, sex, or pregnancy.

But there are also specific physical mechanisms and pathways that contribute to painful sensations during menstruation and other normal reproductive functions, and they have nothing to do with emotions.

The womb (uterus) is not very well equipped with the sensory nerve fibers that convey pain and other sensation messages. Unlike the skin and outer parts of the body, inner organs in general are relatively insensitive (in both sexes) to cutting, tearing, or burning. This is true of the womb, of the inner part of the vagina, and of other reproductive organs too. But the womb does have some sensory nerve endings, and these respond to twisting, stretching, and other mechanical stimuli.

The twisting or stretching of hollow inner organs can be quite painful, as anyone who has ever suffered gas pains or stomach cramps must know. When the womb is dilated or contracted, it sends pain messages to the brain.

What causes the muscle we call the womb to twist, stretch, and contract?

Women's ovaries produce the two sex hormones estrogen and progesterone. These powerful chemical messengers are what make menstruation, ovulation, conception, pregnancy, birth—the whole reproductive process—take place. To accomplish this, they cause things to happen to many organs, including, of course, the womb.

By no means do all women suffer cramps during menstruation. Perhaps the majority never have the smallest menstrual aches. But many women do feel some cramping, especially in the teen-age and young adult years. Some cramps may be caused by emotional problems; a rare few are caused by a disease of the womb or the ovaries. By far most cramping is normal—that is, it is not caused by a disease, physical or mental, and is in fact the result of a normal growing-up process.

Girls start menstruating, at around twelve or thirteen, as a result of the fact that their ovaries have begun to produce estrogen—the primary female sex hormone, and one that their ovaries will produce for the rest of their reproductive lives. It is not until the menopause, occurring on the average at age fifty, that the ovaries will stop producing estrogen and menstruation will therefore cease.

The major aim and function of the menstrual cycle caused by this estrogen is to prepare the lining of the womb for a fertilized egg, which can then develop in nine months into a baby. If the egg is not fertilized, or if no egg has been produced, the lining sloughs off at the end of the cycle—usually about every twenty-eight days—and is discharged through the vagina in the form of menstrual blood.

About midway through each menstrual cycle—around day 14, counting from the first day of bleeding—an egg is produced for fertilization by either of the two ovaries. This process is called ovulation. The egg is produced by a small pocket or follicle in the ovary, and this pocket then develops into a small, temporary gland which produces the other female hormone, progesterone. So in the last half of the cycle, just prior to the next menstrual bleeding period, *both* estrogen *and* progesterone are present in the body.

But ovulation does not happen right away. A girl will normally menstruate at, say, age thirteen, but her ovaries will not begin to produce eggs, will not ovulate, for anywhere from six months to a year or more later. So for this first period of roughly a year, her body is producing *only* estrogen, no progesterone.

Then, suddenly, when she is about fourteen or fifteen, she will begin to ovulate, which means her body will begin to produce progesterone.

Progesterone stimulates the muscular tissues of the womb to stretch and contract. This is something of a hormone shock to the nerve fibers, which are unused to progesterone and its effect and are therefore highly sensitive to it.

Some girls will have little or no discomfort at this beginning of progesterone production. But others will feel a cramplike pain, caused by the reaction of the sensitive nerve endings to the unfamiliar progesterone. Since this progesterone production occurs in the latter half of the menstrual cycle, they will feel the cramps just prior to or at the beginning of their bleeding.

In time this may lessen and go away, as the womb gets used to the progesterone. In some young women it does not go away, and they suffer cramps regularly each menstrual period.

Sometimes a doctor (or a mother) will tell a girl, "Don't worry, it will go away after you've had your first baby." This sounds like a patronizing put-down, and often it is. It is also often true.

Because if a womb is exposed to large doses of progesterone, its nerve fibers do get used to it, become less sensitive, and stop responding to it with pain messages. This is what happens in pregnancy. When an egg is fertilized, menstrual periods stop and the ovary continues for nine months to produce massive amounts of progesterone, which is in fact a pregnancy hormone rather than a sex hormone. The womb gets used to this—in effect gets accustomed to having lots of progesterone around. Most cases of menstrual cramps stop therefore after the first pregnancy.

Because oral contraceptives contain progesterone (as well as estrogen), they mimic pregnancy in a woman's body when she takes them. They relieve menstrual cramps, although that of course is not their chief purpose.

Another painful symptom many women suffer just before menstruation is headache. Sometimes it feels like a migraine. And indeed it is, in the sense that, like migraine, such premenstrual headaches are the result of rapid expansion and contraction of blood vessels in the head.

Estrogen is the guilty party here. This hormone has a powerful effect on blood vessels; one of these is to cause blood vessel expansion and contraction, producing headache not only at menstrual periods but also—because of the sudden rapid decline in estrogen—at the menopause.

A good many migraine headaches occur at the menstrual period, when estrogen levels in the body rise. Migraine sufferers sometimes find that when they take oral contraceptives, their headaches are worse and occur more frequently. And some women who are not migraine sufferers have migraine-like headaches when they take these pills.

The pain of childbirth, probably the oldest pain we know, has nothing to do with hormones, and is caused by purely mechanical actions: stretching, squeezing, twisting, tearing. Here the patient probably knows more about the pain than her doctor.

Women who feel childbirth pain feel it coming at two different stages of labor, from two different locations. First from the cervix, the mouth of the womb, as it stretches to permit the infant's head to move out into the vagina. Sometimes the pressure of the dilating cervix on nearby organs adds to the pain. Second, later in labor, from the opening of the vagina, when these tissues stretch and sometimes tear—and are sometimes cut by the doctor—at delivery itself. Doctors may inject anesthetics at either or both stages to block the pains.

A word about anesthesia, *absence of sensation*, a very different thing from analgesia, *absence of pain*. Local anesthesia is the blocking (deadening) of a sensory nerve fiber's ability to carry messages, including pain messages, from a small (local) area of the body. The anesthetic is a drug that interferes with either the synapses between neurons or the functioning of the neuron itself by temporarily paralyzing the sensory receptor neurons. When local anesthesia is used to cover the wider area, it is sometimes called regional anesthesia. The size of the dose injected into the area to be numbed, or the closeness of the injection to a nerve ganglion, or junction, determines how effective, wide, and long-lasting the anesthetic dose will be.

Injection of anesthetic into each side of the cervix blocks the pain of early-stage labor, when the fetus is pressing against and dilating the cervix, by blocking the nerves. Later in labor injection of anesthetic near the pudendal nerves on each side of the vagina blocks the pain of late labor as the head and shoulders emerge, stretching and sometimes tearing the tissues there. Local anesthetic rarely has any dangerous side effects on the mother, and never on the child.

Spinal anesthesia is injected directly into the spinal column, where the drug bathes the spinal cord. This blocks sensation from all parts of the body below the point of injection, effectively blocking all pain of childbirth. Spinal anesthesia can in relatively rare cases have unwanted side effects on the mother and/or the child.

General anesthesia, which puts the patient to sleep, is the most effective pain-killer. But it influences all systems of the body, not just the nerves, and it has its dangers. Most important, it can result in deprivation of much-needed oxygen for the infant.

The justified fear of anesthesia affecting the baby, as well as the current feeling that one should take as few drugs as possible, has encouraged a trend toward "natural," or nonanesthetic, childbirth. Some young women, depending on their emotional outlook, physical health, and the condition of the unborn baby—and especially its position in the womb—have succeeded in giving birth with little or no anesthesia, feeling little or no serious birth pain. Many others don't mind anesthesia as long as they are conscious and can see and hear their baby as it is born. This can be done under spinal anesthesia, or under regional, local anesthesia.

Cesarean section, delivery of the baby by cutting open the abdomen and the womb, is usually done under general anesthesia. But some physicians have done Cesareans with only local anesthesia, especially when they felt that any stronger anesthetic would be a clear danger to the baby. This kind of birth with only local anesthetic requires great understanding and motivation on the part of the mother. No one who insists on being unconscious for any kind of surgery will tolerate local, regional, or even spinal anesthesia for Cesarean birth.

Dr. Brooks Ranney of the University of South Dakota School of Medicine feels that delivering Cesarean babies under local anesthetic has many advantages. He has delivered 218 babies in this way, and he reports that they breathe and cry much more quickly and effectively than Cesarean babies he has delivered using general or spinal anesthesia. Many of his patients have come back for second, third, and even fourth Cesarean births under local anesthesia.

The technique Dr. Ranney uses is designed to protect the baby when local anesthetic seems safer, as, for example, when the mother has had no medical care during pregnancy and there is reason to believe the baby may need extra help. It is also useful in small, isolated communities where there are not adequate anesthetic facilities or trained anesthesiologists and the doctor performing the delivery has to do everything himself. Dr. Ranney uses the anesthetic drug procaine, first injecting and then cutting, in turn, the skin, the tissues just under the skin, and the lining of the abdomen.

The womb is then opened, the baby is taken out, and the mother is immediately given general anesthesia. Since the baby is born, the anesthesia is no longer any threat. The mother has already seen and heard the baby cry. Now the mother can be sewed up while she is unconscious.

All pains, but especially birth pains, are much influenced by what is going on the the cerebral cortex. No other pain is so strongly affected by emotions, attitudes, memories, and childhood influences as is childbirth pain.

A woman looks at childbirth through the feelings she has been taught about children and motherhood. These feelings influence her response to childbirth pain. Most girls grow up expecting motherhood to hurt somewhat, and indeed it does. A few women are so frightened of what they believe is a special feminine torture that they do suffer extreme pain. These women always need general anesthesia, and they need more of it than other women. At the opposite extreme is the young woman who is bound and determined that she will not feel pain, who is positive about childbirth, and who prepares herself for birth. These young women often succeed in having a "natural," drug-free childbirth.

The woman who suffers terribly should not be dismissed (as she sometimes is) as "being a baby," or "having a low threshold." If she feels pain, it's real; the fact that she screams bloody murder and disturbs the nurses on her floor is no reason to put her down. Nor should the girl who breezes through delivery without a needle or a pill be glorified as a kind of Joan of Arc of obstetrics.

A woman may have different reactions to different child-births, depending on all sorts of varying factors: her general mood, how much she wants *this* baby, her relationship with her husband at *this* time, and so forth. There are women who can have one baby with no anesthesia, and who will need to be knocked out by general anesthesia for another.

Dr. Ranney feels that almost any woman will accept Cesarean delivery with only local anesthesia if the obstetrician first explains to her the advantages to her baby. The knowledge that it is to her infant's benefit, operating through a woman's intelligence, enables her to bear pain.

In addition to deep-seated emotional attitudes, events with emotional impact happening right at the time of delivery can influence the feeling of pain and even the process of labor itself. The entire birth process is a mechanical and inevitable process, governed by hormones, nerve fibers, and muscles that contract and expand involuntarily. But just as the emotion of disgust can ruin a meal, interfere with the normal process of digestion, and provoke nausea and vomiting, emotions can halt the process and sensations of birth.

Dr. Charles Flowers, head of the department of obstetrics and gynecology at the University of Alabama Hospital in Birmingham, tells a story of a woman in the last stages of labor. Suddenly a relative ran into the room to announce that her husband had just died in an automobile accident. The woman's labor stopped immediately and completely. Doctors were able to restart it only by means of artificial hormones after many hours of sleep brought on by sleeping pills.

The same power of emotions over the birth process is seen in wild animals. When a deer about to deliver her fawn is attacked by hunters or animals, she stops in the middle of labor and bounds away to find a safe place. There she resumes giving birth.

Fear or other powerful emotions, operating in the brain, cause the brain to send messages down the nerve fibers to the adrenal glands. These glands then produce a sudden flood of adrenal hormones which stop labor and prepare the body —human or animal—for sudden flight or for other defensive activity. When the individual is relaxed, the adrenal glands slow down to normal and the process of labor resumes.

Chapter 13

Pain and Pleasure

Do people like to be tickled?

They giggle and laugh and seem to behave as if being tickled were great fun.

But they also pull away and cover up their ticklish parts in defensive reflex actions, as if being tickled were painful. Which is it?

Thinking about tickling helps us think about the relationship between pain and pleasure—sometimes opposites, sometime overlapping, occasionally almost identical. Tickling messages, like itching messages, are carried by the same nerve fibers that carry pain messages. It is not until the message gets to the thalamus that it is processed and perceived in the cerebral cortex as tickle, itch, or pain.

Tickling requires a special kind of stimulus—motion. Something—a hair, a feather, a finger—has to move back and forth over the skin, with varying degress of pressure, to create the sensation of tickling. Like an itch, a tickle can be mild, almost pleasant; or it can be torture.

The idea that opposites can be different yet the same is a difficult one to grasp. We see opposites as enemies: truth versus falsehood, good versus evil, light versus darkness, freedom versus slavery.

So with pain and pleasure. We think of them as opposites. Yet our language betrays the confusion that can exist between

114

the two. We describe pleasure as being so intense as to be "unendurable," something we "can't stand." We talk of "exquisite" pain. From the physiological point of view, agony and ecstasy seem remarkably similar.

The ancient Greeks and Romans were very wise about this, despite their lack of anatomic or physiological knowledge about the body. The Roman philosopher Seneca wrote: "There is a certain pleasure which is akin to pain." And Plato describes, centuries earlier, how Socrates, released from his leg chains just before death, scratches and rubs his legs with pleasure. Socrates says: "How singular is the thing called pleasure, and how curiously related to pain, which might be thought to be the opposite of it . . . yet he who pursues either is generally compelled to take the other; their bodies are two but they are joined by a single head."

This concept of pain and pleasure united by a common head or brain comes pretty close to being an accurate image of the nervous system. All sensory nerves feed their signals into a single thalamus, and these are *perceived* as pain or pleasure—sometimes as both.

There are many common examples of mild pain perceived as pleasant, if not as pleasure. Here are some:

1. The tingling that follows a full-force, "bracing" needle shower.
2. The satisfying minor aches and bruises following a game of football or other contact sports.
3. The stimulation of mild blows from twigs or branches, or of a sudden jump into cold water following a hot sauna.
4. Scratching an itch.
5. Coming into a warm house from a snowstorm.
6. Being punched lightly, or squeezed, or bitten lightly, or pummeled, as a show of love or affection.
7. The pain and fatigue of successfully completed effort, as after climbing a difficult mountain.

The list could continue, perhaps indefinitely. And it would be a different list for different individuals—with different pains felt as different pleasures.

In Chapter 3 Dr. Asenath Petrie's theory that there are three types of personalities—reducers, augmentors, and moderates—was described. Reducers, who downplay sensation, were said to be less responsive to pain than augmentors or moderates. They required more sensation than others, and this requirement made them suffer when they were deprived of sensation by solitary confinement in prison.

The discovery that deprivation of sensation is unbearable, is in fact a form of torture, has been widely noted. All individuals, not only so-called reducers, need the impact of sensation to maintain their psychological and physical health. The strange case of Patty Hearst, and her alleged switching over to the side of the Symbionese Liberation Army against her family and her early training, has been described as a case of being "brainwashed."

There is such a thing as brainwashing, and it has been performed, according to the accounts of ex-prisoners, by police authorities in China, Korea, the Soviet Union, and the United Kingdom. British authorities in Ulster have been accused of brainwashing Irish Republican Army suspects or prisoners. In the United States controversial experiments with prisoners in Vacaville State Prison in California (where some of the Symbionese Libration Army people were once imprisoned) have been described as brainwashing.

Putting it simply, the idea of brainwashing is to break down the individual's personality—his or her way of looking at things and of behaving—and creating in the vacuum a new personality to the satisfaction of the captors. The personality is broken down in part by sensory deprivation. Kept in solitary confinement, sometimes in darkness, sometimes in a soundproof room, the victim loses his or her psychological bearings and becomes passive and receptive to the wishes of those in charge.

The body needs sensation. Without it the nervous system, and especially that part of it that is the home of the personality, the cerebral cortex, loses its orientation. The individual loses command of himself or herself, and in the end can actually be permanently damaged.

Under these circumstances, when the *absence* of sensation is like a torture, the *presence* of sensation, even pain, may be a kind of relief from torture, as shown by the adolescent prisoners discussed in Chapter 3 who injured themselves in a desperate effort to feel something—anything.

Any feeling, even pain, is better than no feeling, because it means we are alive. *We feel, therefore, we are*.

Which brings us to that strange mixture of sex and pain we call sadism and masochism, or sadomasochism. The words are combined because of the recent recognition, as Socrates seems to have suggested more than two thousand years ago, that inflicting pain and receiving pain are related. One cannot exist without the other.

Sadism, sexual enjoyment in causing or seeing pain in others, takes its name from the Marquis de Sade, a French aristocrat who wrote about this peculiar "pleasure." Leopold von Sacher-Masoch gave his name to its opposite, masochism, the sexual enjoyment of feeling pain inflicted on oneself.

Oceans of ink and mountains of paper have been used up in an attempt to explain these strange psychological conditions. No one really knows what causes them, or how one can be relieved of them.

But we do know that something *like* masochism and sadism is fairly common among certain animals in our own biologic group, the mammals.

Male cats and lions bite and hold the neck of the female before sexual intercourse. If they do not do this, the sexual act usually cannot be performed.

Male sheep and horses nip and bite the female just before sex. So do seals, rabbits, and some of the higher apes.

Minks, martens, and sable males are so aggressive in sexual activity that it appears as if they were determined to destroy the female. These males bite the female badly along the back of the neck, breaking the skin. If the female does not respond properly—that is, if she does *not* fight back—the male will usually not mate with her. If the male does not "attack" her, the female will not ovulate and, therefore, will not produce any offspring.

This raises a serious problem for mink and sable ranchers, who raise the animals commercially for their expensive furs. If the animals do not fight before sex, they cannot reproduce. On the other hand, if the male gets too rough, he can tear and ruin the female's valuable pelt.

Sex with pain among animals has two important details in common: The male always inflicts the pain on the female, and the pain always serves a purpose. Without this "combat," there can be no mating, because the male or female will not be sufficiently excited. The aggression causes a *physiological* response involving hormones, muscles, and nervous system networks.

In humans sex with pain is entirely psychological, in the mind. It serves no physiological purpose, only the emotional needs of the person concerned. Also, in all human societies in which sex plus pain has been observed, there is a rough equality between males and females: what one does to the other can be done in turnabout—a sort of golden rule, in which neither sex can perform all the sadism while the other accepts all the masochism.

Our own society considers sex an extremely private matter, and so scientists have little useful information on this subject, except to note that a need to hurt or to be hurt is fairly rare. But in other cultures studied by anthropologists, a good deal of rough-and-tumble, rather combative sex has been observed.

In all of these, the pain inflicted in love combat has been mild. It is almost always a matter of hair pulling, scratching, mild biting, or light pummeling. Often it appears to be a kind of "game" in which one partner pretends aggression, and the other pretends resistance. If they really like each other, the end of the "conflict" is predictable.

A certain amount of mild playful pain is combined with sexual excitement in all humans. It is in those rare and strange cases that go past a certain agreed-upon point that it becomes a kind of emotional sickness we call sadism or masochism. How this sickness arises and what it means, no one really knows. Psychiatrists say that it is probably a result of some peculiarity in the early rearing of the individual which somehow connects sex in his or her mind with pain—given or received.

It may be that pain is mixed up in some people's psychology with feelings of power. The greatest power one can imagine is the power to inflict pain on others. Those who need to feel powerful may gratify their needs through sadism. Those who need to feel powerless may have this gratified by submitting, as masochists, to sadists.

Considering not only the vast amount of literature about sadism and masochism but also the enormous popularity of violent acts in movies, television shows, and comic books, we might conclude that there may well be a large amount of sadomasochism in all of us. At least in our fantasies.

Chapter 14

Pain as a
Constant Companion

A doctor's greatest frustration comes when you tell him where it hurts and he cannot help you. Inability to treat pain is medicine's biggest failure.

Unrelieved pain sends sufferers running in desperation to quacks and phony cures. It fills the waiting rooms of so-called miracle workers. It drives others to the abuse of drugs, including legal drugs: alcohol, legal narcotics, sedatives.

How to treat chronic pain—pain that lasts a long time or returns continually over and over again—is a major medical puzzle. Most chronic pain can be relieved, sometimes temporarily, sometimes permanently, by surgery or drugs or some of the newer methods discussed in the later chapters. But the constant use of pain-killers is dangerous. Pain cures may be worse for health than the pain. Drugs and surgery can do permanent damage.

Then there is the special problem of pain that *cannot* be treated—intractable pain.

The problem of chronic or intractable pain is not only one of how to relieve the suffering, important as that is. Pain itself can be a disease, producing symptoms of its own. If it persists, it takes over the sufferer's entire personality, dominating, interfering with work and life.

Constant pain, holding the cerebral cortex in its terrible grip, affects appetite, sleep, blood pressure, and heart rate. It demands all the body's attention and drains all of its energy. Such pain must be treated, or it will prevent its victim from eating, resting, or sleeping. Untreated severe continuous pain will cause loss of weight and strength and will end in physical and mental deterioration.

Somehow one must find a way to live with chronic pain, or one will die of it.

One of the most common of the serious chronic pains is migraine headache. Migraine tends to recur periodically for long stretches, lasting sometimes for a lifetime.

Another common chronic pain is that cause by arthritis, which affects some 2 million Americans, 175,000 of them teen-agers or children. The pain of arthritis is caused by inflammation and irritation of the arthritic joint, and by swelling and pressure on the tendons and ligaments that surround it. When the disease has progressed so far that cartilage in the joint has deteriorated, bone presses against bone. This too can cause severe pain.

An often incapacitating chronic pain is that caused by pressure on the sensory nerve fibers. The friction of bone against nerve, as in the pinching of a nerve root by two vertebrae in back pain, or the squeezing of a smashed arm or leg bone against a nerve, can be excruciating. Even worse is the neuralgia, or nerve pain, that follows certain virus diseases of the nerve fibers. This neuralgia is like a constant burning ache, punctuated by agonizing stabs and flashes. This kind of pain is described by Dr. Melzack as an example of open gate pain caused by destruction or damage to large nonpain fibers. Rubbing the skin helps relieve the pain by sending sensory messages that tend to close the gate. Chronic neuralgia can also be a result of diabetes, anemia, or other diseases affecting nerve fibers.

Probably the most bizarre chronic pain is that of trigeminal neuralgia, or *tic douloureux*. No one knows the cause of this disease. Here is how a medical textbook describes it:

> It is a searing, agonizing stab. . . . Each stab is momentary, but stabs may occur repetitively over periods lasting as long as 20 seconds. Often . . . the stab is initiated by touching a trigger point, which may be on the skin or lips. Even a slight breath of air across the trigger zone may initiate [it].

But the worst of all chronic pain is that of cancer, not only because of its terrible intensity but also because of the emotional impact of knowing that the pain comes from an incurable disease progressing relentlessly to death. Not all cancer kills and not all cancer results in severe pain. Some, like cancer of the brain, may be painless. But cancer is a common and dreaded killer, and the fear it sheds makes cancer pain and its relief a major medical problem.

A cancerous growth causes pain in many ways. It may press against nerve fibers or nerve roots. Or the nerve fibers themselves may be afflicted with the cancer. If one of the body's hollow organs or canals in the urinary or digestive tracts (stomach, bowel, bladder) is blocked by a cancer, the pain is severe. So it is if a blood vessel is blocked or squeezed.

Infection and inflammation resulting from cancerous destruction is another source of cancer pain.

Fear, anxiety, and depression make all pain worse. The knowledge that there is no cure and that death is the usual end makes the cancer patient suffer even more. The reactions he sees in the faces and behavior of his relatives and friends —and sometimes his physician—add to the sum of his pain.

There are some rare cases of chronic pain caused entirely by the emotions. But we need a note of caution when talking about "psychogenic" pain—pain produced apparently by emotional and not at all by physical disease. It is too easy for a physician who cannot find a disease or an injury on which to pin the pain to tell his patient that there is none. The patient then feels he or she suffers from "imaginary" pain, is perhaps a hypochondriac. There are doctors who get rid of patients who complain of constant pain of unknown origin, sometimes by sending them to psychiatrists. Some doctors refer contemptuously to such complainers as "crocks." But it is possible that the pain has a physical cause which the doctor has not been able to find.

This was the case with the young woman with the sinus headache described in Chapter 9. After addiction to pain-killing drugs which led to an attempt at suicide, her psychiatrist suggested risky brain surgery. Fortunately, she consulted a careful surgeon, who was in no hurry to take a knife to her brain.

Until fairly recently the knife was the only alternative to addictive, pain-killing drugs. The pain was relieved by severing connections in the nervous system so that pain messages could not get through to the thalamus and the rest of the brain. These operations ranged from cutting nerve fibers or nerve roots outside the spinal cord, to cutting the cord itself, and even to cutting parts of the brain.

The disadvantages of pain surgery seem to outweigh the advantages. In many cases nerve fibers grow back after the risky surgery, and the pain returns. Or the pain seems to "find" new pathways to get its message through to the thalamus.

Even worse are such results as partial paralysis, loss of sensation in the part of the body involved, and even a peculiar kind of intractable pain surrounded by an area of deadened sensation. Or the pain may be relieved by the surgery, while the patient also loses some control of his or her urination, bowel movements, and other vital processes.

Pain surgery that cuts only the root of the trigeminal nerve fiber often relieves *tic douloureux* without leaving any undesirable side effects.

Cancer pain in patients who are terminal—near death—provides the best reason for pain surgery. The surgery relieves the pain long enough, since the patient's end is near, and the risk of physical harm seems less important than the brief period of release from torture.

But except for specific cases, pain-relief surgery now takes second place to the analgesic drugs.

Chapter 15

Turning Pain Off: Drugs

Drinking, eating, inhaling, or applying a chemical to kill pain is as old as history. Ancient Egyptians and Babylonians used analgesic preparations, some of alcohol, others of opium. South American Indians used (and use) mind-changing drugs made from cactus, mushroom, and coca leaf.

When God performed surgery on Adam and fashioned Eve out of one of his ribs, He used what may have been the first general anesthetic. Genesis says: "And the Lord God caused a deep sleep to fall upon Adam, and he slept."

Today the taking of drugs to relieve pain is so common it is almost universal. Americans spend about $2 billion each year on pain drugs. Such drugs use up a lion's share of television commercial time. They are responsible for many serious health problems in those who overuse them.

Yet despite their dangers, drugs are effective pain-killers and are here to stay. Drug researchers (and drug takers) have to deal with an old pharmacological fact of life: *Drugs that are harmless are useless. The more effective, the greater the risk. There is no such thing as an effective drug that is free of any harmful side effects.*

So it is important to know how a drug works and when to use it. And how not to abuse it.

No one knows exactly how and where pain-killing drugs work, although we do know the ball park they work in.

The most widely used pain-killer is probably aspirin or one of the many drugs in the aspirin family, and for good reason. It is extremely effective against mild or moderate pain, probably the best there is, and has no competition for relieving headache, joint ache, or muscle ache. It even helps relieve toothache, as well as other mild pains. It has other advantages: it is not habit-forming, and has no effect on the brain. It therefore produces none of the dangerous side effects of drowsiness, inattention, or even unconsciousness. With all other analgesic drugs, one risks these dangers.

Aspirin does have its own risks, though. Because it irritates sensitive mucous membrane linings, it irritates the stomach and can cause nausea, vomiting, and stomach pain. It can also cause bleeding of the stomach lining. For both these reasons it is often sold in a combination that includes a chemical buffer that blocks the irritating effect.

Although no one knows for sure, the aspirin family is believed to relieve pain by interfering with the reception of pain signals by the neurons in the part that hurts—head, joints, or muscles. This theory suggests that the chemicals in aspirin-type drugs (the important ones are members of the salicylate family, which takes its name from the Latin term for "willow tree," the original source of aspirin) counteract the chemicals released by injured tissues. It is these chemicals, especially bradykinin, that trigger pain signals in the neuron.

Another theory speculates that aspirin relieves pain by reducing the inflammation that is the source of the pain. Inflammation—swelling, redness, collection of fluids, release of chemicals—is the response of tissue to injury. Aspirin is an excellent anti-inflammatory drug and is the first medicine tried in chronic, painful, inflammatory illnesses such as arthritis. It is of no help in relieving the dull, "deep" pain of the hollow internal organs.

The oldest of analgesic drugs are those in the narcotic family. A narcotic is any drug that in proper doses reduces the ability to feel sensation, relieves pain, and results in sleep, and that in large doses causes unconsciousness and eventually death. Mankind's earliest-discovered narcotic was alcohol. Opium came shortly thereafter, followed by its commonly used derivative morphine.

The term "narcotic" is used today, however, to describe only the drugs that are descended from, or related to, opium, which is made from part of the flower of the poppy plant, and that are regulated by federal antinarcotic law. We speak here only of the *legal* narcotics—those used in medical treatment and available only under a doctor's prescription (with special strict rules governing those prescriptions)—and not of such illegal drugs as opium's other child, heroin, and cocaine. Neither of these last two have any medical value, although they certainly kill pain.

Narcotic drugs—morphine and its relatives—are very effective against severe pain of all kinds, including pain in internal organs. But they are also highly addictive. Problem: How can the sufferer from chronic pain which goes on forever achieve relief without becoming an addict? Answer: He can't, if he takes one of the narcotics continuously. This is their great shortcoming. And this is why, as we shall see in following chapters, the search for nondrug treatment of chronic pain is so important. But so long as they are taken for short periods of time, narcotics are wonderful relievers of severe pain.

The way narcotics work is also a bit of a mystery. It is believed that they work on the brain, probably on the cerebral cortex and the thalamus. They have a specific effect, zeroing in on the perception of pain without having too much influence on the reception of other sensation signals. It is as if the pain is there but is no longer a problem. People describe the effect as, "The pain is still there, but it doesn't hurt."

Because narcotics can produce addiction if taken for too long a time, their greatest value and safest use is in the treatment of short-term pain. This is the kind of pain felt just after surgical operation. Narcotics are also useful for the treatment of the extreme but temporary pains caused by a wound or an accidental injury, or during a kidney-stone attack or other acute pain. "However," says an authoritative medical text-book, "it is tragic when a patient with chronic pain and a normal life expectancy is provided opiates [narcotics]."

For those with a less-than-normal life expectancy, it is sometimes better and kinder to relieve the suffering and forget about the risk of drug addiction. This is the case with terminal patients who are suffering the agonies of cancer and have only months or weeks to live. Narcotic analgesics offer their greatest help here.

There are some less addictive analgesic narcotics, but true to our pharmacological fact of life, they are also less effective. The best known of these is codeine, which is commonly found in cough remedies (it kills the pain of sore throat and the urge to cough) and in analgesics designed to be taken after tooth extraction. Drugs in this family are given for moderate pain that is not relieved by the aspirin family but is not severe enough to require the powerful narcotics. Sometimes codeine is combined with aspirin.

The most commonly used (and abused) legal drugs fall into the family of sedatives, which produce drowsiness, or seda-tive-hypnotics, which produce sleep. (Hypnos was the Greek god of sleep.) The newer members of this family of drugs are sometimes called tranquilizers, but all these mood-changing drugs are basically the same. They are all very widely abused in our pill-popping culture and are generally described as "downers," which is exactly what they do to the body. One of them is said to be the most widely sold prescription drug in the United States.

Although they are often given by doctors for the relief of pain, they are not analgesics, and in fact they may sometimes *increase* pain reactions. And while they are not legally classed as addictive drugs, they can produce addiction. They act like alcohol, which is also a "downer," and just as some (but not all) drinkers become alcoholics, some (but not all) heavy users of these drugs become addicted to them.

These drugs, together with alcohol, depress ("down") important systems of the body, chiefly the central nervous system (including the brain), and the respiratory system, the breathing mechanism. An overdose turns the brain and breathing down, sometimes so far that death is approached and occasionally reached. The body simply stops working.

Less horrifying but more common side effects of sedative-hypnotics are sleepiness, confusion of judgment, and lack of alertness. The drugs act on *all* the sensory-receiving mechanisms, like a shotgun, and do not, like the narcotics, concentrate on the pain-receiving mechanisms.

Then why are they given and taken for pain?

Because they do relieve that part of the pain that is caused or aggravated by the mind, or the cerebral cortex. We know that fear, anxiety, and psychological attitudes contribute to pain perception. By dulling the part of the brain where these emotional forces operate, the sedative-hypnotics reduce the amount of pain felt. Taking sedative-hypnotic pills or drinking liquor does indeed cause one to "feel no pain."

Some of the tranquilizer drugs also reduce pain through another mechanism. These drugs depress not only the brain and the breathing but also affect the muscles attached to bone and skeleton. They are, then, muscle relaxants, and the reduction in muscle tension they produce lessens the pain caused by such tension, especially headache and backache.

Any discussion of analgesic drugs has to include some mention of a surprisingly powerful one—the placebo! A placebo is really a *nothing* drug, a make-believe used to fool the sufferer into thinking he or she is really being given a medicine when in fact it is only a "sugar" pill, an injection of water, or a tablet of some harmless, useless, inactive chemical.

Placebos work. In one campus experiment conducted by

Dr. H. K. Beecher—the man who discovered that wounded soldiers on Anzio felt no pain when they knew they would be sent home from the war—morphine was compared with a placebo. Some patients suffering severe pain were given morphine, and others were given the nothing drug without being told that it was a placebo. Thirty-five percent of the patients who were given the placebo of sugar or salt reported relief of their pain! Such is the power of the mind over pain. Placebos are said to work in about one-third of all cases.

We have been talking about analgesics, which block only pain, and not about anesthetics, which block *all* feeling. But sometimes local anesthetics are useful for analgesic purposes. This is especially the case with the chronic pain from neuralgia or pain from certain kinds of cancer. The local anesthetic, often procaine or lidocaine or another of the "caine" family, is injected in and around the particular nerve fiber carrying the pain signals. The actual chemical effect of the drug lasts only for hours, but in many cases the pain does not return for days and even weeks. In some special cases nerve fibers can be destroyed by injection of neurolytic (nerve-killing) drugs, so that pain is gone for months and even longer.

In our overmedicated society more and more people are becoming aware of the risks of drug taking. No one really knows what effect the constant swallowing or injecting of powerful chemicals is having on the body. Thus the search for newer and more precisely targeted pain-killers goes on, helped along by the light thrown by the gate control hypothesis.

Chapter 16

Jamming the Pain Signal: Electroanalgesia

The failures of the knife and the dangers of pills have led pain doctors to experiment in the last few years with electricity. The Melzack-Wall hypothesis encouraged them to attempt to block pain signals by sending electric charges along the fast nonpain nerve fibers to close the pain gate. This so-called electroanalgesia, one of the children of gate control theory, is, like its mother, a source of enthusiastic disagreement.

Not that electrical pain-killing is so new. Thousands of years ago Greeks and other ancient peoples used electric fish to relieve pain—probably not electric eels because they put out almost five times as much voltage as standard household current. A Roman physician in the year A.D. 46 described using electric fish for treatment of headache. The fish was held against the aching head until it numbed the pain away.

If one accepts the gate idea, the principle of electrical pain-killing is simple. A charge is delivered to the spinal cord by means of the fast nonpain nerve fibers. Getting there long before the pain signal, the electric signal, which feels like a buzzing or vibrating, stimulates the substantia gelatinosa cells to close the gate.

Electroanalgesia can be accomplished in three ways. In the simplest and now most commonly used approach, electrodes are placed on the skin close to where it hurts. Batteries send pulses of current to the electrodes. The current is picked up by the fast fibers and carried to the spinal cord.

A slightly more complicated method for deeper pain requires surgical implantation of the electrodes under the surface of the skin right on the nerve fiber that is carrying the pain to be treated. This is done under local anesthesia; at the same time a receiver is implanted just under the skin at a convenient spot near the electrodes. The electrodes and the receiver are connected under the skin by fine wires. A small battery-operated stimulator provides the current. Its electrodes are placed on the skin just above the receiver, and the current is then sent to the electrode on the nerve being treated.

Even more complicated, hazardous, and controversial is the implantation of electrodes under general anesthesia inside the spinal column around the rear of the spinal cord. The receivers are placed under the skin below the collar bone, and a wire traveling inside the body passes from the receiver over the shoulder and down the back to the electrode.

In any of these techniques, the patient may get a small carrying case for his stimulator. He can then send gate-closing messages to relieve pain at any time or place, wherever he may be.

Electroanalgesia works with *some* patients. It relieves *some* kinds of pain. It is especially useful in treating chronic pain from cancer, neuralgia, and a phantom limb. It seems to relieve acute pain at the incision following certain types of surgery.

The fact that electroanalgesia works doesn't prove that the gate theory is correct, any more than the fact the fire walkers of Sunderpur could walk on hot coals proves that the goddess Kali protected them. No one really knows *how* electric charges relieve pain or *where* the charges do this. Or why in some cases electroanalgesia doesn't work at all. It has yet to be proved that the substantia gelatinosa cells function as Dr. Melzack believes.

Electroanalgesia does suggest to some pain researchers that the gate theory is, in general, correct. Others disagree, as we shall see after we take a look at some actual cases of pain relieving.

Dr. Alan Hymes, assistant clinical professor of surgery at the University of Minnesota, used a device powered with flashlight batteries (4.5 volts) and connected to electrodes taped on the skin. This electric current relieved severe pain right after chest and abdominal surgery. The electrodes were placed as close to the wound as possible. (See Figure 7.)

This pain-killing device was tried on 230 patients right after the surgery. The majority of them had some relief from pain, and as a group, they suffered fewer complications than did

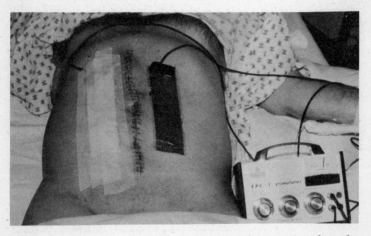

Figure 7. An electric device in place to relieve pain after abdominal surgery. The electrodes are taped onto the skin on each side of the incision.

Photo courtesy Alan Hymes.

other patients who did not receive electrical stimulation. The chest surgery patients who received it had only one sixth as many lung complications as the others. Only one of the abdominal surgery patients (less than 1 percent; there were 170) had temporary paralysis of the bowel. But 13 percent of the patients *not* receiving electrical stimulation *did* have bowel problems.

How does Dr. Hymes explain the *why* of electroanalgesia? And how does he explain its reduction of complications?

"It may be in part explained by the Melzack-Wall hypothesis concerning gate control," said Dr. Hymes.

But I personally think that hypothesis doesn't explain many of the details of our observations. And I attribute the low proportion of complications to the fact that reduction of pain allows patients to take deep breaths and cough, and this helps prevent lung problems following chest and abdominal surgery. With regard to the bowels in the patients having abdominal surgery, in my opinion the elctrical current seems to have some direct effect stimulating the bowels to function.

Dr. Hymes reports that both groups of patients were able to leave the intensive care units one day earlier than the usual average stay.

Minneapolis, where Dr. Hymes lives and works, has been one of the centers of research on the use of electricity to relieve pain. Some of the earliest success stories have been reported from that city.

One Minneapolis housewife reported that the little electronic box she carried around and used periodically to block her pain signals changed her life from torture to joy. "I had terrible back pains for seven years," she told a newspaper reporter. She said she had spent close to one thousand dollars on drugs that simply dulled her awareness without relieving her pain.

Then Dr. Don Long, one of the pioneers in electrical pain relief and now at The Johns Hopkins University, where he is director of the department of neurosurgery, provided her with the electroanalgesia device. The woman simply tapes electrodes about the size of a silver dollar to her back. Wires connect the electrodes to the box where she controls the current. At first she had to use the box continuously, but after six months she found she had to use it for less than an hour each day. The current causes no unpleasant sensation, only a slight tingling on her skin. The only problems so far with this skin surface electroanalgesia has been slight irritation, redness, and blistering of the skin in some users.

Only two firms make the devices, and both are located in Minneapolis. The box, plus carrying case, wires, and electrodes, sells for about two hundred dollars. It weighs three pounds and is about as big as a medium-sized transistor radio.

At one time Dr. Long was one of only three physicians in the country who had any experience with electroanalgesia. Now there are a few more, but still not very many. Dr. Long has done implants of spinal column electrodes as well as implants under the skin near a nerve fiber. He reports many difficulties and failures with the electrodes placed near the spinal cord, but considerable success with those placed under the skin around one of the outer nerve fibers.

Dr. Long did this for ten people suffering from various kinds of nerve injury pain, implanting the electrodes on the nerve close to the location of the pain, mostly in arms and legs. This brought complete pain relief to six of the ten and partial relief to two. In one patient the electric charge did not relieve the pain, and in one it made the pain worse.

Nine of the patients had become addicted to pain-killing drugs. After electrical stimulation, seven of them completely kicked the drug habit.

To the question: "Does your success with electroanalgesia

prove that the Melzack-Wall theory is correct?" Dr. Long answers: "The simple fact that the electrical stimulation seems to work for pain does not corroborate the gate theory. It suggests that the gate theory may be correct in a general way, but does not support its localization in the substantia gelatinosa in the spinal cord."

The first successful treatment of pain by electricity was done in 1967 by Dr. C. Norman Shealy of the Pain Rehabilitation Center in La Crosse, Wisconsin, and he did it by implanting electrodes around the spinal cord. Dr. Shealy got the idea from the Melzack-Wall hypothesis, which was published two years earlier.

But for some patients the electricity hurt more than the pain, so Dr. Shealy began trying to find out in advance which patients were suited for electroanalgesia and which were not. One of the testing methods he used was to place electrodes on the surface of the skin near the pain and to see if a test charge worked. This is how Dr. Hymes' and Dr. Long's electroanalgesia approach, which is now the more commonly used, was born.

But first Dr. Shealy and others performed many spinal cord implants, finding that the method worked for some kinds of pain and for some patients, but not for all. Today such implantation is used less and less at Dr. Shealy's pain clinic, and he has come to feel that chronic pain is more often influenced by habit and emotional responses—that it is, in fact, best treated psychologically. Over 80 percent of the chronic pain patients at the Pain Rehabilitation Center now are treated by psychological means.

Some of the bad results with implanting electrodes on or near the spinal cord have only recently been reported. As with any new cure, the first few years of electroanalgesia were filled with reports of sensational success. Now, eight years after Dr. Shealy's first successful implant, the failures are beginning to turn up with greater frequency.

One case reported in early 1974 described a woman who had an electrode implanted for relief of chronic back pain. It worked for six months, and then suddenly the pain came back. Then a year later additional excruciating pain developed in the back of her neck, and the right side of her body became paralyzed. An operation was performed to look at the electrode, and a hematoma, a kind of blood blister, was found to have developed under it, pressing against the spinal cord.

In a similar case described by Dr. Arthur Taub of Yale, one of the early pioneers in pain mechanism research, an electrode placed over the spinal cord produced no relief of pain at all when it was activated. But it did cause cramps and muscular spasms in the legs of the patient, a fifty-three-year-old man, as well as loss of control over his urine and other signs of beginning paralysis, including numbness of the lower half of his body. When the current was turned off, these signs cleared up, but only gradually.

Dr. Taub is one of the most outspoken critics of both electrical stimulation of the spinal cord as used for analgesia, and the gate control hypothesis. He cites reports of dangerous side effects, and he thinks that there is much indiscriminate use of implanting of electrodes either on the peripheral nerves or on the spinal cord. He suggests that in some cases where electrodes seem to work it is because they do possibly irreparable damage to some part of the nervous system. He believes that thus far electrical stimulation of the skin alone works no better than a placebo, except when nerve endings are directly anesthetized.

His chief objection to the gate theory is that he believes the evidence advanced for it is weak and indirect. "No one knows what the function of the substantia gelatinosa is," he says,

and none of the cells in this part of the spinal cord have ever been studied thoroughly and carefully. Most of the cells and systems of the theory are purely hypothetical.

There are other important details in the hypothesis which to me aren't supported by convincing information, such as the idea that the role of small fibers is primarily to open previously closed gates.

Despite Dr. Shealy's disillusion, Dr. Taub's opposition, and recurrent reports of failure, a growing number of physicians, like Dr. Hymes in Minneapolis, are reporting success with surface electroanalgesia. And Dr. Long remains optimistic. He finds it most useful in treating, not severe chronic pain, but less serious, more acute pains.

And he does not agree at all that the use of electroanalgesia has been indiscriminate. "The development of these devices has been handled very well. Electrical stimulation has probably been used on the most highly selected group of patients, and has been carefully controlled.

"As contrast, I would point out the flurry of activity around acupuncture, where little control has been exercised."

This brings us to the Chinese connection in the new wide-open field of pain-killing.

Chapter 17

The Chinese Connection: Acupuncture Analgesia

If using mild electric shocks to block pain is something of a puzzle, sticking needles into people to block pain seems like something out of a horror movie. And yet it is said to work —sometimes.

In discussing and evaluating acupuncture analgesia (and acupuncture anesthesia), we are at some disadvantage. Most of the experience with it has been in China. Although some American (and other foreign) physicians have gone to China and reported on what they saw there, not all the background details about the patients and their preparation for the analgesia or about long-term aftereffects were available to them. And these are essential to evaluate such a procedure. Second-hand reports, even by trained investigators with all the facts at hand, cannot take the place of direct observation of experiments done under carefully controlled circumstances.

Such careful studies have been done on electroanalgesia, as Dr. Long has pointed out. As he also pointed out, the use of acupuncture in this country has been haphazard and sometimes careless.

Following President Nixon's visit to China an enormous interest in all things Chinese, including acupuncture, caught the public's attention. As is so often the case with a new and sensational medical practice, particularly one that promises the as yet impossible—a simple, harmless, "perfect" method of relief from chronic pain—a number of so-called acupuncture clinics staffed by "acupuncturists" suddenly appeared. Some of these seemed eager and willing to separate patients from their dollars, if not from their pain. Some states and the District of Columbia permit acupuncture by non-MDs. The classified advertisement shown in Figure 8 makes claims not made by Chinese acupuncturists and not supported by reliable scientific data.

Yet there is a solid body of information that suggests that acupuncture may someday earn itself a respectable place in American medicine. Much of this information comes from China by way of American medical experts who have visited that country and have examined Chinese medical care as guests of the China Medical Association.

MEDICAL ACUPUNCTURE
for CHRONIC PAIN

Due to Arthritis, Bursitis, Neuralgia, Neuritis, Back Pains, Muscle Spasms, Sciatica, Tics, Paralysis, Paresis, Tennis Elbow, Shingles, early M.S., Torticollis, Asthma, Peptic Ulcers, High Blood Pressure, Insomnia, Sinus Problems, Colitis, etc.

and
PERSISTENT HEADACHES
NERVE DEAFNESS & Tinnitus
SEXUAL DYSFUNCTIONS

Free information provided as a public service. Write to:
Medical Acupuncture Foundation, (non-profit)
99 Highland Av., Somerville, MA. 02145, or call (617) 354-6363

Figure 8. An advertisement in a Boston newspaper.

Courtesy American Medical Association.

The use of needles to treat medical problems has been part of Chinese folk medicine for at least two thousand years and probably longer. But the use of it *to block pain in surgery* is only ten to fifteen years old. Chinese physicians who have been trained in Western medical science use and believe in acupuncture analgesia or anesthesia but are *not* strong supporters of acupuncture for other purposes.

Since 1971, when a group of prominent American doctors headed by E. Grey Dimond and the late Paul Dudley White returned from China with their firsthand reports of major operations performed under acupuncture, world medicine has paid respectful attention to this as yet unexplainable pain-killer. They and later American medical visitors have witnessed and described operations on the thyroid gland, the stomach, the lung, and other internal organs. Except for a mild dose of a narcotic analgesic during the surgery and a sleeping pill the night before, the only anesthesia used in these operations, all of which are performed in the United States under general anesthesia, was acupuncture.

The acupuncturist either twirled the needles slightly after they were inserted or delivered a low electric charge—about 9 volts—to the needles by a small battery source similar to that used in this country for electroanalgesia. During the operation the patient was cheerful and conscious, and in some cases he got off the operating table and left the room under his own power after the surgery!

The description of an operation for removal of a kidney stone especially interested me because I have recently had the same operation, done in New York under general anesthesia. The Chinese patient, a man about my own age, had a much better time of it according to Dr. H. Len Tseng.

Dr. Tseng is chief of anatomical pathology at St. Elizabeth's Hospital in Washington, D.C. He described what he saw in China in an American medical publication.

The man with the kidney stone was given a sleeping pill the night before. Half an hour before the operation, two long needles were inserted in his right side—that's the side the stone was on—two more in his forehead, and then two more in the tip of his nose. The six needles were then connected to an electric box producing 9 volts of continuous current. That's about as much current as three two-battery flashlights. The only medication given the man was a light dose of Demerol, a narcotic analgesic, injected into his veins.

"The whole operation," Dr. Tseng writes, "lasted approximately 40 minutes. . . . I conversed with the patient during the entire operation. He was never unable to answer my questions clearly; he even smiled on several occasions."

Compared to my own experience, which was in all other respects successful, this Chinese kidney-stone patient had an easy time of it. General anesthesia, for those who have never undergone it and don't know what it's like, is almost as bad as the pain it relieves. My operation took at least an hour and a half (I can't remember) and was followed by considerable nausea and discomfort for at least a day. I don't believe I was able to "smile" and "answer questions clearly."

One of the most spectacular things about acupuncture is where the needles are inserted. This seems to have no relationship at all to the pain. It is one of the most puzzling facts of acupuncture, and the one that leads many otherwise open-minded scientists to be suspicious.

For example: For an operation in which the chest is cut open and a portion of diseased lung cut away, one needle was inserted between wrist and elbow. An operation for removal of the stomach was carried out with four needles inserted into each earlobe. For a thyroid operation one needle was inserted in each arm.

Acupuncture surgery has also been done occasionally in this country. In Boston's Beth Israel Hospital a young woman had her appendix removed under acupuncture anesthesia, the first such operation done in the United States. It required eleven needles and small amounts of sedative and narcotic analgesic drugs. Newspaper reports said that she was able to walk out of the operating room following the surgery.

Other reports of needles used for analgesic purposes have not been so positive, especially when they were done at so-called acupuncture clinics. Doctors at the University of Virginia Medical Center recently described in the *Journal of the American Medical Association* six patients who had gone to local acupuncture clinics for relief of pain, and had then had to be treated in nearby hospitals for the results of the acupuncture! Among these unlooked-for results were infection caused by unsterilized needles and puncture of internal organs.

Why the Chinese reports describe great success while the few American reports do not has not yet been explained. It may be because American acupuncturists lack the skill and training of the Chinese. Or it may be because of different attitudes and expectations on the part of American patients. This bring us to the most puzzling question of all: How does acupuncture block pain?

One theory, put forth by those who are unimpressed with the technique, is that it works for the same reason that walking on fire is possible for some Indians: the faith of the patient. In other words, the power of the mind over pain. Brought up in a culture that believes in acupuncture, Chinese expect it to work, and in fact it does—for them. (Not all Chinese surgery, by the way, is performed under acupuncture anesthesia, only about 20 to 30 percent. The rest is done under conventional anesthesia, as in this country. Patients may choose either method.)

It has also been claimed that acupuncture works psychologically, through hypnosis. But hypnosis usually requires prolonged training on the part of the patient. When hypnosis is used for surgery here, the hypnotist usually needs from four to eight hours to put the patient into a deep enough trance.

Furthermore, only about one person in five can be hypnotized. Yet a much higher proportion of Chinese patients are said to respond to acupuncture.

Probably, the most telling argument against the hypnosis explanation is the fact that animals' pain can be blocked by acupuncture, and yet they are not subject to hypnosis as we know it, nor are infants. "The anesthetic effect [of acupuncture]," says Dr. H. Jack Geiger of the School of Medicine, State University of New York, Stony Brook, who visited China and observed acupuncture surgery there, "is *not* due to any kind of hypnosis, unless one is willing to accept the unlikely proposition that horses, mules, cats, rabbits, and human infants are susceptible to hypnosis."

There is also a traditional Chinese folklore explanation, based on the concept of Yin (the spirit) and Yang (the blood). According to this belief, which is contradicted by modern anatomy and physiology, Yin and Yang are carried in channels of the body, and the acupuncture points lie along these channels and the places where they intersect.

Some modern pain experts think that the traditional acupuncture points may be at places where sensory and motor nerve fibers lie just below the surface of the skin, so that piercing them with needles, especially when the needles are then charged with electricity, has an effect similar to that of electroanalgesia.

Another explanation, this one coming out of Chinese research laboratories, is that fluids surrounding nerve cells may be involved. These fluids, basically water plus such chemicals as sodium and potassium, play an important part in the synapse transmission of nerve messages from one neuron to another. There have been reports from China of spinal fluid from an acupunctured rabbit blocking pain when it was injected into the spinal column of another rabbit.

Modern Chinese researchers tend to believe that acupuncture blocks pain by sending sensory nonpain messages to the spinal cord and thence to the thalamus and cerebral cortex. "We think," the chief researcher of the Shanghai Institute of Physiology told Dr. Geiger, "that any kind of sensory impulse can inhibit pain to some extent, but only those arising from the site of acupuncture are most effective."

That sounds very much like the Melzack-Wall gate control hypothesis. Dr. Melzack naturally agrees that his hypothesis probably plays a part in explaining acupuncture. But he does not overlook the other explanations:

> My personal opinion is that the mechanisms are as follows. The patients' faith in the procedure as a result of long cultural experience, together with the explicit suggestion that the patient will feel no pain, greatly diminishes anxiety from the outset. Mild analgesic drugs would have the further effect of making the acupuncture procedure more tolerable. . . . The sensory stimulation itself would then activate brainstem areas that block signals which are produced by the surgeon's knife.

Dr. Melzack adds, "This explanation is pure conjecture," and he goes on to place his hope for an answer in future research.

Such research is proceeding here and in China. In 1973 the *Chinese Medical Journal*, now available in this country with English-language abstracts of its scientific papers, reported experiments on forty-five guinea pigs. The animals' responses to pain were blocked by acupuncture. The scientists were looking for that part of the brainstem that might be the location of the blocking. Another paper reported the suggestion that the relationship between large and small nerve fibers may be behind such blocking.

In the same year the National Institutes of Health called a meeting of twenty-six medical schools and universities to discuss acupuncture research in this country. The conference decided that well-designed, carefully controlled studies of this new method of pain-killing should be performed and evaluated before it is used widely on patients.

A number of such experimental studies are now going on. One project at Emory University in Atlanta is trying to determine if there is any neurophysiological basis for acupuncture anesthesia. At the University of North Carolina another study is testing the ability of acupuncture to alter the sensation of touch and the sensations of heat and vibration in the skin.

Until such research has provided final answers to the many questions raised by acupuncture, it should be considered an experimental method to be used in laboratory studies and other scientific projects and not on patients. This is the opinion, following a careful study of acupuncture in China and in this country, of Dr. John J. Bonica, chairman of the department of anesthesiology at the University of Washington and an eminent researcher in pain and its treatment. It is shared by most pain experts.

Chapter 18

Mind Over Pain: Hypnosis and Biofeedback

Pain begins and ends in the mind. It is, therefore, only natural that the newest efforts to control chronic pain should concentrate on the all-powerful cerebral cortex.

We know that pain hurts more when we constantly think about it, when it frightens us, when we are depressed, and when we are tense. What is new, startling, and full of promise for chronic pain sufferers is the fact that these can be controlled by the person in pain—not through drugs or other outside forms of treatment, but by the power of the mind alone.

The oldest method of mind control is hypnosis, misnamed because hypnosis does not really mean being put to sleep. What it does mean is more like *daydreaming*.

Hypnotism is not something a hypnotist does to you but something you do to yourself under his teaching and guidance. So the fact that one can or cannot be hypnotized—and only about one person in five can be—is not a reflection of the skill of the hypnotist but of the kind of person one is. Most people who can be hypnotized can learn to do it to themselves; some don't even need a teacher.

The best way to explain it is not by the word "sleep" or "trance" but by the word "attention." Under hypnotism one's attention is powerfully concentrated, focused, we might say,

on a single particular thing or subject, away from the many
stimuli that bombard us during normal consciousness. It is
this intense concentration on one specific thought or thing
that gives a hypnotized person the appearance of being "in a
trance."

Hypnotism for the relief of pain focuses one's attention
away from the pain. The subject just puts the pain out of his or
her mind. It is as if the hypnotized cerebral cortex were saying to the pain signals coming in from the spinal cord and the
thalamus, "Don't bother me now, I've something else on my
mind."

How it works no one knows, exactly, but work it does for
some. Of the one in five who can be hypnotized, a few can be
anesthetized sufficiently to undergo major surgery with no
drugs or other analgesic preparation. The majority of
hypnotizable individuals, while unable to do without some
anesthesia, require less during surgery than the rest of us.

Those gifted people who can hypnotize themselves are apparently able to turn their pain off as if by an act of will.
For such people chronic pain presents less of a problem. They
need not risk crippling surgery, addictive drugs, or other
risky methods of pain relief. They can continue to live and
work successfully even though they are burdened with pain
that would destroy others.

There have even been cases of individuals who have suffered terrible and painful accidental injury and have been able
to hypnotize themselves sufficiently to get themselves to a
hospital for medical treatment.

But few of us are so fortunate, although some hypnosis
experts claim that the majority of us are. Perhaps it depends
on how sick one is; how much one is suffering, and how
desperate one is.

We need not speculate on one detail concerning hypnosis,
and this is the capability of the mind to turn its attention away
from pain and therefore not to "feel" it. Dr. Ernest R. Hilgard

of Stanford University, a psychologist who has done much research in hypnosis, reported the results of an interesting experiment to a meeting of the American Association for the Advancement of Science early in 1974.

Dr. Hilgard performed experiments with volunteers who were subjected to two kinds of pain: pain produced by placing the hand and arm in ice water, and pain produced by blocking blood flow in an arm by means of a tourniquet. The volunteers experienced these kinds of pain before and during hypnosis, and then they reported how severe the pain was. "Pain reduction," said Dr. Hilgard, reporting his results, "depends on degree of hypnotizability, with highly hypnotizable subjects feeling no pain at all."

But what was most interesting about this experiment was his finding that "some part of the hypnotized person may actually feel the pain that is denied." Dr. Hilgard used a technique he called automatic talking to find out what the "hidden observer," as he called it, had to say about the pain, while the person studied seemed to be unaware of any suffering.

While the subject was hypnotized, and before the pain began, Dr. Hilgard said:

> When I place my hand on your shoulder, I shall be able to talk to a hidden part of you that knows things that are going on in your body, things that are unknown to the part of you to which I am now talking. The part to which I am now talking will not know what you are telling me or even that you are talking. When I remove my hand from your shoulder your memories will be just as they are now.

When his hand was on their shoulder, the subjects reported more pain than when his hand was not on their shoulder, and less pain than when they were *not* hypnotized. The "hidden observer" said that the water was very cold, but it didn't really hurt. And this "observer" reported that pain from blocking blood flow was severe, *but that it didn't hurt.*

Dr. Hilgard thinks that hypnosis produces a kind of amnesia to pain. "A special kind of amnesia in which the pain is blocked from awareness by an amnesia-like process before it has ever come to awareness." He adds, "I do not wish to suggest that we understand this process."

"Biofeedback"—a word invented in 1969—is the newest mind-operated technique for controlling pain. Actually, it's based on controlling those of the body's involuntary processes, such as blood flow and internal muscle contraction, that contribute to pain.

When I was a biology student, we were taught that the so-called involuntary actions of the body—breathing, heart rate, blood pressure, blood flow, digestive functions—were under the control not of the "intelligent" cerebral cortex but of the "stupid" (mindless) autonomic (sympathetic) nervous system. We were also taught that this nervous system is regulated by the bottom-most tip of the brainstem.

So it is normally, except that we know now, only in the past few years, that human beings can be trained to control the "uncontrollable" life processes solely by *thinking* about them—or by *not* thinking about them.

Biofeedback occurs when a person learns how to "listen" to his silent bodily processes, detect when they are going too far in one direction (muscles too tight, too much blood flow to head), and then feeds that information back into his body. He "thinks" his involuntary processes back to where he wants them. This, of course, means that they are no longer entirely involuntary but are somewhat under the control of his will.

The process is very much like yoga. A trained yogi can control his blood pressure, heartbeat, respiration, and many other normally involuntary processes. But *he* does this only after much training and long experience in meditation —another term for focusing the mind inward, on one's internal processes, away from outside stimuli—while most people can be trained to use biofeedback. So say biofeedback experimenters at Topeka's famous Menninger Clinic.

Biofeedback to control pain has so far been successful only in treating migraine and tension headaches. The discovery of its relationship to migraine came about accidentally.

A few years ago doctors at the Menninger Clinic were performing experiments on blood flow and other involuntary processes. A woman volunteer was being trained to control blood flow in her hands, as measured by hand-skin temperature.

During the training the woman suffered an attack of migraine. *But she suddenly recovered at exactly the same time that the temperature in her hand rose ten degrees in two minutes, indicating a sudden increase of blood flow into her hand.*

When word of this spread through the clinic, two other individuals who were migraine sufferers volunteered for training in control of hand temperature. One was entirely successful, the other partly successful in relieving the migraine.

And so the experiment on migraine was begun.

Seventy-five patients, sixty-three with migraine, the others with tension headaches, were told how to use a "temperature trainer," which measured the temperature difference between a finger and the center of the forehead.

They were also provided with a list of certain autogenic (arising from within) phrases to learn: "I feel quite relaxed." "My arms and hands are heavy and warm." "I feel quiet." "My whole body is relaxed, and my hands are warm." "My hands are warm." "Warmth is flowing into my hands."

The patients were told to think about the phrases while they watched the temperature trainer. If the temperature of the hand went up, they knew they were concentrating properly. If it did not, they concentrated harder.

At first they used the trainer every day and reported to the physician in charge once or twice a week. Then they used the trainer only on alternate days. After a month they no longer needed the trainer, but were able to raise hand temperature almost at will, just by thinking "warm" thoughts.

But the best test was the fact that three fourths of the migraine sufferers (not as many of the tension headache patients) were able to relieve their migraine pain. It was important, however, that they begin thinking about hand warming at the *outset* of the migraine attack, before it got under way.

Dr. Joseph D. Sargent of the Menninger Clinic, leader of the team that has been experimenting with biofeedback hand warming, says that those who learn how can increase their hand temperature in less than a minute, but that it must be done just prior to the beginning of a migraine attack. "The most difficult situation," he says, "is when the patient has already begun a moderately severe to severe headache. The reason is probably that the person cannot relax and focus his attention sufficiently while suffering with an intense headache."

Dr. Seymour Diamond, who is president of the American Association for the Study of Headache and the National Migraine Foundation, feels that training in hand warming works best with young migraine sufferers. "It seldom helps anyone over thirty," he says. "But I have about eighteen young patients who can actually abort their migraine headaches."

Hand warming doesn't help tension headaches, but another form of biofeedback does: learning to control muscle spasm. Tension headache is caused by continual contraction of the scalp, neck, and forehead muscles, and the biofeedback used here is one of "plugging in" to these.

Dr. Thomas H. Budzynski of the University of Colorado Medical Center trains tension headache patients to "listen" to their forehead muscle, which is the most important one in headache, by means of an electromyograph (EMG). This instrument records muscle response to electric charges, much as an electrocardiograph records the heart's responses. The leads of the EMG are taped to the forehead, and the instrument is hooked up to a set of earphones.

The patient lies on a bed while he or she wears the earphones, which produce a tone whenever the frontalis (forehead) muscle contracts. The higher the muscle tension, the higher the pitch, and the patient tries to keep the pitch as low as possible. He or she does this by relaxing, by putting all thoughts out of mind, and by concentrating on keeping the tone low. Average biofeedback training consisted of twice-weekly twenty-minute sessions, plus twice a day sessions at home without the equipment.

Dr. Budzynski found that eventually the headache sufferers learned to control the frontalis muscles simply by an effort of mind, without having to use the EMG and earphones. As a result, they were able to feed back their relaxation thoughts to their forehead muscles and thus relieve or even avert tension headaches. He claims that about three-fourths of those he has worked with have been treated successfully by this biofeedback method. Other doctors report similar successes.

Biofeedback in the relief of pain (and in other forms of medical treatment) still has a long way to go. Its application in relieving and treating tension and migraine headache pain is the most successful and best researched of all its uses. This success holds out great promise of developing mind-centered techniques for relieving other chronic pain.

Chapter 19

Pain and Purpose

The ancient Greek god-hero Prometheus was the creator and befriender of mankind.

When he saw that his "children" were cold, miserable, and in darkness, he resolved to steal fire from the gods on Mount Olympus and make a present of it to mortals. This is one version of how man discovered fire.

But Zeus, ruler of the gods on Olympus, was so angry at this act of rebellion that he sent two giants to capture Prometheus and chain him to the top of Mount Caucasus. And there he lay, bound in chains, for thousands of years. Zeus also sent a giant eagle (in some versions of the myth a vulture) to tear and eat Prometheus' liver!

The pain was eternal—chronic—as well as terrible. Although the eagle devoured the liver each day, at night it regenerated itself and grew back. There was no end to the pain.

But there could have been.

If Prometheus had submitted, had given the fire back, and had agreed that Zeus was lord and master of all creation, the eagle would have been sent away, and Prometheus would have been unbound. If he had complained, if he had prayed to Zeus, his pain would have been ended.

Surrender was his morphine, his anesthetic, his electro-analgesia, acupuncture, and biofeedback. He disdained them. His pride and integrity helped him bear the pain so that humanity would have fire and, in effect, some freedom from the tyranny of the gods. He saw a purpose to his pain.

A thousand years passed before Hercules came, broke Prometheus' chains, and killed the eagle. Prometheus then made peace with Zeus, but on his own terms, and for his own purpose. Humanity kept fire.

In Dr. Melzack's gate control terms, if we see a purpose to our pain, our cerebral cortex sends messages down the cord which tend to inhibit our perception of the pain. Purpose closes the gate.

Pain is part of life, and sometimes it has purpose. It warns us of injury. It is the companion of much that we do. It begins our existence and joins us again at its end. Most acute pain is bearable, with analgesic help. Healthy people prefer to *feel*, rather than to live a life of no feeling, a life of anesthesia.

But, on the other hand, there is nothing sacred about chronic pain; it has no merit in and of itself. And it often has no purpose at all. When it takes on a life of its own, when it is persistent and permanent, when it enslaves and torments, it must be defeated.

The trick is to win the battle against pain without losing one's sense of life, one's ability to feel. There is no easy answer, no magic, perfect pain-killer.

Nor will there be. Hercules will not come and free us, because we are men and women, not god-heroes.

INDEX